GARY S. HITZIG, M.D., with twenty years of experience in combating hair loss, is a widely published innovator in the field. He has appeared on major TV shows, including "Donahue," "Good Day New York," CBS TV, NBC TV, "People Are Talking," and Long Island News TV Tonight and on radio. His work has been highlighted in major magazines and newspapers across the country, including *Men's Health*, *GQ*, *Business Week*, *Crain's*, *The New York Times*, *The New York Post*, *USA Today*, *Philadelphia Inquirer*, and *The Boston Herald*. Dr. Hitzig lives on Long Island and practices on Long Island, in New York City and in New Jersey.

HELP & HOPE FOR HAIR LOSS

GARY S. HITZIG, M.D.

AVON BOOKS NEW YORK

The ideas, procedures, and suggestions in this book are intended to supplement, not replace, the medical advice of a trained medical professional. All matters regarding your health require medical supervision. Consult your physician before adopting the suggestions in this book. The author and publisher disclaim any liability arising directly or indirectly from the use of this book.

Excerpt from "The History of Minoxidil" reprinted by permission of the publisher from Gerald R. Zins, Ph.D., *Clinics of Dermatology*, October-December, pages 132 and 198, copyright © 1988 by Elsevier Science Inc.

AVON BOOKS
A division of
The Hearst Corporation
1350 Avenue of the Americas
New York, New York 10019

Published by arrangement with the author
Visit our website at **http://AvonBooks.com**
Library of Congress Catalog Card Number: 96-95173
ISBN: 0-380-78710-5

First Avon Books Printing: May 1997

Printed in the U.S.A.

RAI 10 9 8 7 6 5 4 3 2 1

To Sue, Ben, Carly, Porschia and Sugar Hitzig
(the last two are mutts)—
thank God for all of you!

ACKNOWLEDGMENTS

No finished book is written by just the author. Help comes in many forms from the people who guided his early experiences to those who have been a part of his professional and often personal life. This is no exception.

I need to thank several people here: my wife, Suzanne, for her constant support, feedback, and talented illustrations in this book, and who made the overwhelming do-able for me; Seymour Handler, M.D., my long-term partner and brother-in-law—it's been quite a lifetime; John Schwinning, M.D., my patient, my partner, and a skilled surgeon who is helping bring hair replacement surgery into the next century; Louis Amico, my twenty-year office administrator, confidant, advisor, and best of all friend; Stephen S. Power, my editor and my ultimate teacher of Write from Wrong—his sharp mind and insight shaped my thinking and this book, his belief in me made this happen; Kim Ruben, her administrative, organizational, and typing skills kept pace with an often difficult and demanding author—thank you, Kim; Paul Goldberg, M.D. and Michael Kassouf, M.D., whose skills and devotion helped pick up the slack while I was busy researching and writing; Ron Kirk and Steve Fitzgerald for searching out the proper pictures to illustrate my points and for always being there for me; Walter Lozano, the military lost a good man to me—your skilled mind and hands would be a shame to waste; Steve Archibald, Linda Morgan, Wilfredo Martinez, Dr. Jim Malecka, Derek Nicolls, Marvin Wilson, Angela Wan, Albert Wan, Ron Rivers, Charles Neuls, Jeannette Melendez, and Christine Woods. You are the best staff this one doctor could ever ask for; and finally, my heredity (Sol and Florence Hitzig)—without your genes I never would have lost the hair that propelled me into this field.

There hath not come a razor upon mine head. . . . If I be shaven, then my strength will go from me and I shall become weak, and become like any other man. . . . She made him sleep upon her knees and she called for a man, and she caused him to shave off the seven locks of his head; and she began to afflict him, and his strength went from him.

—Judges 16:16–19

CONTENTS

PREFACE

This book is on a subject which I take very personally. I wish it existed when I was a young adult because I lost my hair when I was eighteen years old. I'll never forget "friends" asking me if I planned to park cars in the "alleyways" on my head and if my hair was stiff enough (God bless hair spray) to knock nails into wood. My hair loss continued rapidly as I got older and thus I needed to investigate possible remedies.

Perhaps like yourself, I investigated the 1970's versions of lotions, potions (not dissimilar from the ones today), and even scalp injections all in an effort to save my wavy locks. As a result, and I hope unlike you, I blew all my earnings from five summers on useless remedies. Finally I was referred to a Manhattan doctor to have hair transplants. This seemed legitimate and the answer to my prayers. Unfortunately, they weren't very good and to cover that disfigurement I wound up with a hairpiece (and a severe depression).

One Sunday morning I was walking down York Avenue in Manhattan with a young lady. We were on our way to brunch when a gust of wind blew my wig off. Another woman, who was walking toward us, was so startled that she spilled her bag of groceries all over the sidewalk, and

I ran out of sheer embarrassment. I never saw my date again. I stopped dating and started exploring other possibilities.

In 1975, when I was a surgical resident at Memorial Sloan Kettering Institute in New York City, I met an attending surgeon undergoing a hair transplant (my wig still covered mine). Thinking I would eventually refer him to my wig maker, I waited and watched his progress—he looked very good. He introduced me to the surgeon who had performed his hair transplant and I began undergoing repair. The surgeon saw my keen focus on hair and invited me to assist him and learn the technique. I traveled the country and to Europe to learn my trade and all I could about hair. My life in hair loss and its replacement began.

I've probably performed more hair replacement surgery than anyone in the world—over thirty thousand procedures—and have advised more than three times as many patients over the years. I lecture to both doctors and the lay public worldwide and continuously engage in research to help improve the plight of the person suffering from hair loss. My publications have increased exponentially and I've just patented my first invention—all in an effort to help remove the stigma of being bald from men and women. I have been on over three hundred talk shows both on national T.V. and radio and have been interviewed by the news media over a hundred times concerning hair loss. With every patient I talk to or perform surgery on, I've never forgotten the daily embarrassment and despair I suffered and finally cured. I love patients guessing my age as ten years younger; and although I exercise extensively, I will always believe it's because I now have, again, a full head of hair.

More important, I can also report that I'm happily married with two wonderful children.

So I dedicate this book to all of us with hair loss and the quest for its remedies. May this book answer your questions and help guide you to your appropriate solution, for "a knowledgeable consumer is his own best friend."

G. S. H

INTRODUCTION

Did you know that 70 percent of all men and 20 percent of all women will experience significant hair loss in their lifetime? If you're one of the victims, these percentages may offer you some comfort (misery enjoys company) but I hope to offer you more by answering your questions regarding the three "C"s of hair loss.

CAUSE

CHOICES (of treatment)

CURE

First, I will answer the most important question, "Why am I losing my hair?", in order to help you understand the various causes of balding.

From here we journey through the psychology of hair loss in order to answer the question inevitably asked next, "Why me?"

Once you understand the causes, we will explore what your hairstylist can do to help, and which of the vast number of nonsurgical treatments are of value. This book will try to steer you away from the scams and let you understand which treatments are good, bad, and useless.

You certainly should have a lot of questions about medications such as Rogaine™ (minoxidil) and Proscar; I will answer these for you. In doing so, I hope to help you understand the benefits and limitations of each before you spend a lot of your hard-earned money purchasing them. I'll also show what the future of drug therapy holds for us.

If you don't want a medical treatment, then you may want a hairpiece or system. We'll see what they are, what they cost, and what their strengths and weaknesses are.

If you want a permanent solution to your hair loss problem, then you will need to enter the vast and confusing world of hair loss surgery. No one considers this option without asking many questions. Having lost my hair has enabled me to know the questions that you would and should ask and my vast experience and research will help answer them for you. You'll learn all you need to know about transplants, scalp reductions, expanders, extenders, flaps, suture methods, cloning, and the surgical procedures of the future.

There may be questions you have that are not touched on here or not fully explained to your satisfaction. In these cases you should seek the proper professional guidance. This book will also offer you a blueprint to finding the right ethical professionals to deliver sound, reliable answers.

ONE

"WHY AM I LOSING MY HAIR?" (AND WHEN SHOULD I START TREATING IT?)

When I was seventeen and starting losing my hair I went to see a dermatologist. He told me worry was the enemy of the scalp—so I shouldn't worry. Naturally, this made me worry more and I lost my hair.

Anonymous patient

During fetal development, hair can be found all over the body. At birth, the newborn is surrounded by vellus or very fine hair which remains as such on various parts of the body for life. As the baby gets older, various vellus hairs become what we call true hair (terminal or thicker pigmented hair), and this is what we grow on our childhood and adult scalps. Male and female pattern hair loss (or androgenetic hair loss) involves the reversion of true hairs back to the almost invisible vellus hair. This is what most of us refer to as hair loss, but this is not the only cause of hair loss, just the most common.

The causes of hair loss have been categorized in more

recent years and are described in detail below. Knowing which applies to you is your best chance of finding the right solution.

WHAT IS MALE PATTERN BALDNESS?

Fifty percent of men suffer noticeable hair loss by age fifty. It characteristically appears after the onset of puberty and peaks in the twenty-one to forty-five age group. The patterns and types of loss have been charted by both Dr. James Hamilton (a full professor of anatomy at the State University of New York, Downstate Medical Center, and my anatomy teacher in medical school) and Dr. O'tar Norwood, a dermatologist with extensive research and publications in hair loss.

NORWOOD HAIR LOSS CLASSIFICATIONS

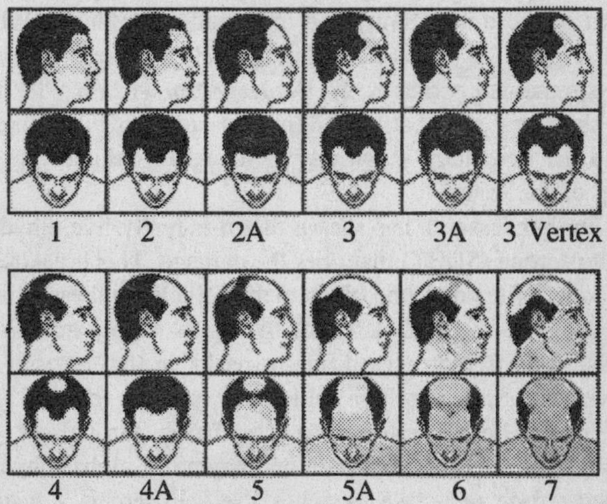

O'tar Norwood, M.D.

It can begin in the crown (monk's cap) or in the front and can progress to complete (not the sides or back) hair loss on top.

WHAT ROLE DOES TESTOSTERONE PLAY IN MALE PATTERN BALDNESS?

Dr. Hamilton once told me how he discovered the cause of male pattern baldness.

There was a singing group in Italy called the castrata. These were young males castrated prior to puberty to preserve their soprano voices. Oddly enough, none of them suffered male pattern baldness. Dr. Hamilton decided to experiment on a group of volunteer castrata. He administered testosterone to them in various dosages to bring their male hormone levels to normal. He noticed roughly 65 percent of these men developed male pattern baldness. When he stopped the testosterone, guess what happened—the hair loss remained permanently. Dr. Hamilton was thus the first to show that male pattern baldness is caused by testosterone and the hereditary sensitivity to it of hair follicles on the top of the scalp.

Further research has shown that it is really five dihydrotestosterone (5DHT) that does the damage. This breakdown product of testosterone binds to the follicles and essentially destroys them by choking off the blood supply and nutrients. At different ages different peaks in the testosterone level will cause sensitive follicles to involute (die).

Here's how: Testosterone circulating throughout the body has receptors to which an enzyme, 5 alpha dihydrotestosterone reductase, attaches itself. (There is a natural attraction for enzymes and receptor sites to combine in all of us.) When this happens, the enzyme allows the conversion of regular circulating testosterone to dihydrotestosterone, 5DHT.

Further experiments were performed to see if people who did not lose their hair had receptor sites for the 5 alpha dihydrotestosterone reductase. At first, investigators felt that perhaps it was the lack of sites that allowed people to keep their hair. But deeper investigation proved that all scalp hairs have sites for the enzyme. This then allowed the further conclusion that only hair follicles whose genetic code allowed the dihydrotestosterone to choke off the blood and nutrient supply would react negatively to the 5DHT. In fact it soon became evident that the 5DHT affected only scalp hair and not body hair at all.

Later experimentation actually showed a difference in testosterone metabolism (breakdown) between scalps destined to have hair loss and those that would keep a full head of growing hair upon it. In essence, these later results confirmed that male pattern hair loss is dependent on hair root sensitivity to various levels of 5DHT although other factors are still being investigated.

WHAT ROLE DOES GENETICS PLAY IN MALE PATTERN BALDNESS?

Another interesting aspect of male hair loss has to do with the inheritance of the gene for baldness. Not that many years ago we were taught that genetic hair loss was sex linked and thereby transmitted from the mother's side only. We have since learned that this was only the tip of the iceberg. Like a political investigation, as the research goes deeper, more and more players (in our case, chromosomes) are implicated. Although male pattern baldness is definitely transmitted on the X chromosome (XY is a male, XX is a female), there are numerous other chromosomes (humans have forty-six) that help determine the age of occurrence, rate, and degree of hair loss. So just because your maternal grandfather is bald doesn't mean you will be also.

WHAT ROLE DOES STRESS PLAY IN MALE PATTERN BALDNESS?

We now know that stress can speed up the rate of hair loss. Although it usually does not cause permanent loss in an area not meant to bald, it can considerably move up the time frame in which genetically doomed hair dies. I saw this in a patient who came to me after completing a crash diet of 140 pounds in a six-month period. He virtually starved himself, but he was desperate to lose the weight. During that same period he had also lost most of the hair in the crown area of the scalp. He was quite distressed by this because he felt his effort to look good was now being sabotaged. When I told him that severe stress in any form, be it psychological or social, can cause a speed-up in the hereditary hair loss process, he became depressed. After working with him psychologically as well as surgically, we restored his hair and his confidence. And yes, the weight remained off.

Stresses such as the loss of a loved one can similarly speed up hair loss. I have witnessed this many times. Physical stress such as heavy athletic training as well as even the simple stress of moving to a new country with a new language can push the fast forward button on male pattern hair loss. So when I think of the doctor who told me that stress was the enemy of the scalp, I would have to guess here that he was not all wrong. We'll discuss the treatments later. For now it's important to understand that stress can help cause hair loss other than that determined by heredity. We see this in alopecia areata (described below) as well as other more dramatic forms of baldness, such as that which occurs during chemotherapy. What is important to remember is that with the exception of hereditary and exotic causes for balding, hair will generally grow back.

When a male patient asks me how I know his hair loss is genetic, I usually tell him that there is little else that will cause a man to lose the hair from the top of his head but spare the hair on the sides and back. Although the crazy myths that we will explore later may seem logical to the male victim of balding, simple reasoning will help him get back on track.

WHAT IS FEMALE HEREDITARY BALDNESS?

Yes, women suffer hereditary hair loss as well and it's time doctors and patients realize this is a common problem for which treatment, not shame, should be encouraged. We know that 15–20 percent of women will suffer enough hair loss in their lifetime as to cause a noticeable thinning. All women have both female (estrogen) and male (testosterone) hormones in their system. The loss or lowering of the protective estrogen allows the testosterone to exert its effect on hair follicles, causing a thinning (or veil effect) of the hair on the top of the scalp. Women rarely suffer shiny bald areas and almost always only have a noticeable thinning; however, enough women reported this problem to their physicians that classification of female pattern baldness (not unlike the male counterpart) occurred as far back as 1974.

Sometimes the first evidence of genetic hair loss in a female is the widening of her part, whether it is the center or on the side. In this case the usual thin, often whitish, scalp that is normally visible expands on each side, making the part more of a zone. In general the hairs that will become extinct are not all grouped together, but are instead interspersed between active growing hairs. This is what creates the veil effect so often seen in this pattern, which allows us to see through the thinning hair.

WHAT ROLE DOES TESTOSTERONE PLAY IN FEMALE PATTERN BALDNESS?

Women as well as men have the enzyme 5 alpha reductase present in the scalp region. This, as with the male model, acts to convert the available testosterone to 5 dihydrotestosterone (5DHT), the culprit in genetic balding. In Japan, a researcher, Dr. Sawaya, in the late 1980's and early 1990's showed, however, that women have an additional protective enzyme (aromatase) which helps block the conversion of the testosterone to 5DHT. Finally in women, as well as men, there is much higher 5 alpha reductase activity in the front of the scalp as compared to the crown region, thereby increasing the likelihood of thinning in the more noticeable frontal section near the hairline.

WHAT ROLE DOES ESTROGEN PLAY IN FEMALE PATTERN BALDNESS?

The onset of female pattern baldness most commonly occurs during menopause when the woman begins to lose the "protective" effects of estrogen. But this is not the only time that it can occur. Although there may be other influencing factors, we do know that anything, be it drug or event, that alters the protective levels of estrogens can lead to an earlier development of female hair loss. This is not unlike the stressful causes of premature male balding mentioned earlier. It is not uncommon for me to see a female patient in her late twenties who comes in after several frustrating years of varying her hairstyle to cover her thinning hair. More tragically I have seen several young women who had hairpieces either woven or glued to thinning areas which accomplished nothing more than to cause additional, and in several cases severe, permanent hair loss. This is because we know that scalp inflammation leads to a greater vulnerability of the hair follicles to 5DHT and thus an earlier demise.

One cause of premature hair loss is birth control pills. Because hormonal balance is being immediately manipulated, permanent hair loss can and does occur. I have also seen young women who have lost quite a bit of hair after pregnancy when their hormonal balances were readjusting themselves. Although I have seen several women who regrew much of their hair, I have seen even more who did not.

WHY DO SOME WOMEN SUFFER HAIR LOSS AFTER SURGERY?

Some women have come to me complaining of early permanent hair loss after surgery. At first I couldn't connect it, but all of them seemed to have a family history positive for female pattern balding. When I took a further careful history, I found that all of them had general anesthesia and all of them had the same anesthetic agents (halothane and ethrane). The *Physicians Desk Reference* didn't seem to support this as a cause and I can only hypothesize that it was a combination of the stress of general anesthesia coupled with some unknown effect of these two agents that caused the early expression of female pattern hair loss.

CAN MEDICAL TREATMENTS AND GENETICS INTERACT?

A great deal of additional research needs to be conducted in all areas of genetic balding, but none requires more than the female pattern and its expression. It is an investigation whose time has come. I recently saw an eighteen-year-old female college student who had very thin hair in the front of her scalp. It was so thin, in fact, that her college "friends" would brutally tease her by claiming that she had some disease. She became socially withdrawn and soon her grades began to show it. Her mom brought her in and I could find no positive reason for hair loss in her medical history. Her mother had thinning hair but it hadn't occurred until she was in her late forties. She later called me after they left to tell me she had been on birth control pills but couldn't say so in front of her mother (and her prior medical evaluation never mentioned it).

This taught me a valuable lesson. When it comes to interviewing prospective patients (as they are interviewing me) during an initial consultation, I must make attempts to learn additional valuable history from the potential patient that he or she may be too shy to repeat with a friend or relative in the room. This has been as true over the years with parents and their offspring as it has been between husband and wife. I will never forget how amazed I was when I was talking to a husband and wife once. She made her husband leave the room before she would remove her hairpiece. It seemed that he had *never* seen her without it, and today was no exception.

So now after talking with a duo of either parent and child, husband and wife, or boyfriend and girlfriend, I will make the effort to contact the patient later in order to get any additional history I need. I also once had a woman who came in with her spouse and who swore to me that she was evaluated by prior doctors and told she had hereditary hair loss. She wanted a transplant, no ifs, ands, or buts. When I called her at work she was so surprised at my questions that she then felt it necessary to tell me the truth; she had lied about all prior evaluations. It turned out she had hyperthyroidism (a fast thyroid) as I had thought when I examined her. I thought this because all of her scalp hair was thin, not just that on the top of the head.

So please tell the truth to your doctor. Your honest answers will enable your doctor to treat you best. You wouldn't want to fool yourself into surgery, I'm sure.

WHAT ARE THE OTHER CAUSES OF HAIR LOSS?

Tricotillomania

This is a condition affecting both man and beast (we see it in nervous French poodles and African Grey parrots). In the human form, a person constantly twirls his hair with one hand while either talking, reading, writing, etc., causing an inflammatory reaction at the hair follicle from the constant tugging and ripping. Subsequently this causes permanent hair loss in an uneven random pattern. This can occur in any hair-bearing area. I remember one patient who was sitting there twirling his hair out of nervousness while he was denying to me that he did it. I wound up asking my assistant to snap a Polaroid when he wasn't looking and showed it to him; what a surprise!

Animals cause the same result by biting and ripping out their fur or feathers. For example, African Grey parrots will rip out most of their feathers if they suffer a separation anxiety from their owner, leaving a bald talking bird. This topic leads us to the next and somewhat related category.

Traction Hair Loss

Tight braiding or cornrowing hair (such as Bo Derek's hairstyle in *10*) over a prolonged period of time causes the same result as tricotillomania, that is, inflammation and eventual death of the hair follicle. I can't tell you how many African-American women present themselves to me after extensive hair loss (which is too often permanent), seeking a solution they wouldn't need if they had prior knowledge of the damage they were causing.

This is also the case in various types of prosthetic hair

replacements where hairpieces or tufts of hair are attached for long periods of time to the person's own existing hair. It is especially true in hair weaving where braids of the person's own hair are used to attach a larger hairpiece unit to it. Tightening the hairpiece to the braids causes continuous traction. Similarly, in bonding, where hairpiece systems are glued directly to the person's remaining hair, any motion or manipulation of the system exerts traction on the living hairs of the scalp that are covered by the unit. Hair extensions where tufts of hair are added to the person's own remaining hair by tying them together will also cause added traction stress.

I have seen other more exotic prosthetic additions using Velcro and snaps for the connection. Remember, anytime you use remaining good hair to anchor a larger piece or system, the added weight will cause a level of traction proportional to the weight and size of the addition. Too often I see a patient with circular patches of permanent hair loss in areas where clips or braids were applied in an effort to anchor a hairpiece. These are generally permanent areas of hair loss and do not regrow when the piece is removed even for an extended period of time.

This cause is much more common than you would at first think. All too often I see a young lady (or gentleman) come into the office with a hairpiece on. When they remove it, I nearly gasp. You see, the hair loss from long-term braiding occurs in any area of the scalp and therefore potential donor area for transplantation can be destroyed. Sometimes the damage is so severe, as I saw in one thirty-two-year-old woman, that I had nothing to offer the patient. It is gut-wrenching to face a patient who cries hysterically over something you have no power to help. She told me that if her parents found out what she had caused (they had warned her) they would disown her. I reassured her that her parents sounded loving and would support her through this, and fortunately I was right. She wound up with a custom hairpiece through which her remaining hair was integrated. She still had worries when dating (because she was single and quite attractive), but she eventually found her Prince Charming.

Other people cause permanent traction hair loss with poorly attached hairpieces or wigs glued onto remaining hair. There is no quick fix for hair loss but there is quick damage to remaining hair. You must be so careful in all aspects of hair care and hair replacement; the consequences can be devastating.

Alopecia Areata and Totalis (Universalis)

Alopecia areata is thought to be an autoimmune reaction where the body actually attacks itself, destroying the hair follicles. The condition is probably stress-related and causes circular patchy areas of hair loss. We saw this on Mike Tyson early in his career in the front of his scalp as well as on Roger Maris in 1961 during his drive to beat Babe Ruth's home run record. This was widely reported in the press that year.

Generally, whether it is treated or not, hair growth will return in less than six months but it can be recurrent and, in some cases, if the hair hasn't returned after a year, there is a good chance the damage is permanent.

Although various forms of medical treatment are available to aid the hair in regrowing, there is certainly no guarantee. Areas where hair is permanently lost can and have been successfully transplanted so the condition is not as hopeless as it may sound. Of course, transplanting hair requires areas of healthy growing hair to use as a donor and this is certainly not available in alopecia universalis. In any case, please see a physician regarding your hair loss. Delays can be very costly.

Alopecia areata is not by any means a rare condition. There is a National Alopecia Areata Foundation that answers over ten thousand separate inquiries per year. Each year they also supply a video to over two thousand children to help them explain alopecia areata to their schoolmates. Their services do not stop here. They maintain direct contact with over five thousand people who have needed the support services that they provide.

In an effort to educate the public and those who are afflicted to the diagnosis, problems, and consequences of alopecia areata, the foundation runs an annual conference. In recent years over seven hundred people attended this conference. This is a staggering figure as most major medical conferences generally have less than two hundred attendees.

The foundation also runs a summer camp/conference for kids and teens with the disease, and has a consistent attendance of over 150 children.

Scholarships and grants are awarded to needy patients and innovative researchers respectively. Grants in recent years have amounted to hundreds of thousands of dollars, all of which are the product of private fund-raising. Their active public affairs section has been successful in placing over one hundred publicity pieces in magazines, newspapers, radio, and television annually. See the resources section at the end of this book for more information on the National Alopecia Areata Foundation.

Alopecia totalis is the extreme version of the above where all body hair is completely lost. This is usually permanent and traumatic to the patient.

Chemical Hair Loss

So you decide you'll look better by perming or straightening your hair. As I see too often in my practice, numerous people go to a person with little or no experience, or decide to save money and "do it themselves." You must know the pitfalls. I had one young lady who came to see me. When I asked what was the problem, she handed me a plastic bag filled with hair. When she took her hat off, I saw where it once was. She was crying hysterically but managed to tell me that she had asked a friend to "straighten" her hair. The friend used plenty of chemicals, thinking more is better. What she didn't realize is that many straighteners contain lye and other caustic chemicals. These can produce a chemical burn resulting in destruction of the hair follicle. The same is true with the newer chemical straighteners and with perms.

Similarly I've had patients bring in labeled bags of hair showing me the day and amount of hair that fell out. They should have seen me right after the first bag. Early treatment can help prevent permanent hair loss but is no guarantee.

Be careful!

Drugs

Various drugs can cause a usually temporary hair loss of the scalp. Some of these are

- amphetamines
- anticoagulants such as Coumadin and high doses of aspirin

- overactive hyperthyroid medicines slowing thyroid function and thus causing hair loss
- chemotherapy for cancer
- antidepressant drugs such as lithium
- oral contraceptives, as well as some drugs treating high blood pressure such as Hydrodiuril and Captopril

I had one female patient who was treating her acne with Retin A and Accutane and had her hair thin at the same time. She came to me to see if she should get her acne back, thinking it would help her hair. I'll never forget her statement, "I'd rather have pimples than look freaky." She changed medicines and her hair regrew. Always check with your doctor and pharmacist as to the possible side effects of any medication you are about to take.

Diseases

Various imbalances such as fast or slow thyroid function (hyper or hypo thyroid) can significantly thin the hair. Medical treatment usually corrects this by returning your thyroid hormone production to its normal rate.

Infections

These can cause scalp scarring and thus permanent hair loss. They range from fungal, viral, and bacterial topical infections (i.e., ringworm) to body-affecting diseases such as syphilis.

Yes, George Washington, who died of syphilis, was bald and wore a hairpiece.

Burns

Both physical and chemical can do it. For example, I treated a fourteen-year-old who had acid spilled on his head on the New York subway. His mother brought him to see me because he was suspended from school because he wouldn't remove his hat nor tell the principal why. He's back in school now and with no need for a hat. I performed two scalp reductions on him which eliminated over 95 percent of the bald area, allowing him to once again comb his hair normally and appear as if he never had the problem.

Miscellaneous

There are some more obscure reasons for hair loss, such as radiation or malignant tumor cells on the scalp. Whenever hair loss occurs it's always best to have a physician examine your scalp in person.

WHAT WILL NOT CAUSE HAIR LOSS?

I could write a book (another one) just talking about the excuses patients have given me for losing their hair.

- No, hats do not cause hair loss even if they are football helmets.
- Going into the military and having your head shaved doesn't do it either.
- Decreased blood flow to the scalp will not cause it. (You have more than you need.)
- Neither does poor diet.

- Nor does lack of vitamins or minerals.
- No, your hair follicles are not getting clogged, causing your hair to continue growing under the scalp until you use some miracle drug to release them.
- Losing your hair is not an allergic reaction to your pet.
- Working in a dusty environment will not cause hair loss.
- Smoking may be linked to lung cancer, but it is not linked to baldness.
- Baldness is not a punishment for not leading a righteous life.
- It is not a result of brushing your hair with a stiff hairbrush too often.

If you have others—please drop me a line. I may use it in my next book.

WHEN SHOULD I DO SOMETHING ABOUT MY HAIR LOSS? AS SOON AS IT BOTHERS YOU!

Several years ago, I conducted a survey of over five hundred patients of all ages (the oldest was an eighty-one-year old widower who wanted hair so he could look better and date younger widows in their sixties). The results showed the following.

- Younger men (and women) are most affected by hair loss because of peer concerns and the social pressures of dating (remember I was one!). Some younger patients (in their early twenties) actually stopped dating and others dropped out of school because of ridicule from peers. This group should have guidance and treatment as soon as possible. Some young people I've seen haven't really gone bald but only had the mild hair recession normal of adulthood. Others wind up losing a lot of money on fake cures and scams.

- Police and firefighters seek help the soonest and in the largest numbers because of a macho image and increased numbers of peers joking about hair loss. They also wear hats which mess hair and make thinning areas harder to conceal when the hats are removed. They are constantly reminded of any balding condition by their colleagues.
- Many people did not seek assistance because of either refusal to admit the problem to themselves, embarrassment in people noticing a sudden change in their appearance, or fear of hair replacement surgery.
- 75 percent received their initial advice from a non-medical "consultant" and 55 percent of patients wished they sought medical advice sooner.
- After the 1987 market crash, many executives used their severence pay to improve their appearance before reentering the job market.

WHO SHOULD I SEE?

Your first step is to see your own physician. If he is not knowledgeable about hair loss, he should refer you to a physician who specializes in this field. Make sure the doctor has not only years of experience, but keeps current in his field by going to seminars and conferences focused on hair loss and its treatment.

He may diagnose genetic (male pattern) baldness. In certain difficult or odd cases we may refer you to an experienced dermatologist for further tests.

Most importantly, ask questions of your physician pertaining to his qualifications and experience in the field, about the treatment alternatives he is presenting to you, and the cost of each. You should feel comfortable with the answers. Second opinions certainly can help. It would have saved me years of misdiagnoses and bad treatment causing both emotional and financial headaches had I sought a second opinion sooner.

WHAT QUESTIONS SHOULD I ASK?

Some important ones are

1. How long have you been in this field and how many procedures have you performed?
2. Have you published articles or lectured on hair loss and treatments for it?
3. Do you go to medical meetings about hair loss each year?
4. Have you treated many people with hair loss?
5. Why are you bald? (If applicable.)
6. Why am I losing my hair?
7. What tests do I need to help nail down the cause?
8. What medical or surgical treatments are available to me?
9. Am I a good candidate for any treatments and why?

10. Can you give me long-term followup on the treatments?
11. Do you have any written information?
12. Do you have any patients like myself that I can talk with?
13. Do you have before and after photos? (If surgery is an option.)
14. Are there any groups or organizations that can give me additional information?
15. What is the cost of your suggested treatments?
16. Can you explain how you arrive at the charges?
17. Are there any additional charges (for example, for followup visits or suture removals)?
18. What are the payment terms?

Most Important: Do not try to diagnose or treat yourself!

You can always call the American Academy of Cosmetic Surgery (312-527-6713), the American Hair Loss Council (312-321-5128), or the American Society for Dermatologic Surgery (800-441-2737) for an appropriate referral to a qualified physician in your area.

TWO

WHY ME?
THE PSYCHOLOGY OF HAIR LOSS

HOW DO MEN SUFFER PSYCHOLOGICALLY?

Most men have similar hair loss experiences. An otherwise healthy young male is suddenly faced with a gradual yet dramatic change in his appearance for, he believes, the worse. This change is progressive and permanent. The dilemma is compounded by the fact that socially and historically it is unmanly for a male to be concerned about his appearance.

Thus conflicted, many men suffer tremendous anxiety about their hair loss. They are on one hand depressed about the appearance and stigma of baldness and on the other hand they are often ashamed to admit that the condition bothers them for fear they would be considered vain. So many men try to compensate physically, psychologically, and socially. They often manage by secretly trying to cover up their bald spots.

For example, when I first began performing hair transplants I sat down with the owner of a large construction company for a consultation. He immediately told me he was very successful. He went on to say that he gets up in the morning, exercises (he was in good shape), showers, and puts on very expensive clothing. But no matter what he spends on clothing and accessories, when he glances in the mirror, he "still looked like crap." This was because he was bald and trying to comb his hair to hide it. He was only succeeding in becoming depressed.

Similarly, when I first started losing my hair, I would keep lowering my part to cover more and more area and it became an obsession. My patients today confirm that they too could spend upwards of one or two hours per day trying to cover what nature was removing. Others seek hope in the opposite route. They shave everything. But nothing can help escape the fact that they are losing their hair.

And if hair loss is traumatic for men, it's devastating for women.

HOW DO WOMEN SUFFER PSYCHOLOGICALLY?

In the past women often avoided discussing hair loss with anyone but their hairdressers. Because they most often suffer from a diffuse thinning, it was generally easy to disguise the problem. But women were nonetheless disturbed by it. They tell me now that they feared detection because, although it was normal for men to lose hair, female hair thinning was considered unnatural, a sign of some disease process.

However, women are becoming much more open about this perfectly ordinary problem. In the 1970's I treated one female patient every two to three months. I now talk to and treat two or three weekly.

I had one patient, Linda R., who refused to leave her

house. When she was forced to, she wouldn't go anywhere without a hat. She stopped attending family functions and wound up on antidepressants. Post-transplant, Linda began appearing with me on national T.V. shows. Ladies' magazines began to write about her and her experience, and soon females with hair loss began to seek help.

WHAT ARE THE PSYCHOLOGICAL PHASES MEN AND WOMEN EXPERIENCE?

When their hair begins to thin, both men and women go through the same psychological phases that follow the loss of anything or anyone dear to us (hair is certainly up there on the list). These are as follows:

DENIAL
PANIC
ANGER
WITHDRAWAL AND DEPRESSION
ACCEPTANCE AND RESOLUTION

CAN THIS REALLY BE HAPPENING TO ME?

Denial

No one wants to believe that this is really happening to themselves. The early hair loss sufferer sees a change in his hair, the temples are receding, or the crown seems a bit thin, but he denies the obvious. He checks the shower drain, comb, or hairbrush (I did) and then looks at his scalp under the brightest and dimmest of lights. He or she carefully listens for comments from others and then reviews all available photos of themselves from second grade onward to see if it's really true. The new sufferer studies his relatives and carefully asks questions about their hair loss, looking for discreet differences between himself and his genetics. This strategy only works for so long. Sooner or later the thinning increases or a "sensitive" friend points out his increasingly visible scalp at a social gathering. Every time he talks to someone their eyes seem to travel to his vanishing hairline.

When you begin to realize the inevitable, it's time to go on to phase two. When I began to lose my hair, I was only seventeen. I first thought that I was brushing it too hard, pulling it and causing it to break. Soon I had my parents' photo albums out on the table end to end when no one was home. I went out in the wind to see if it looked thin when windblown, and I would wet my hair and carefully look for telltale scalp in the bathroom mirror.

Most of all, like in any pending loss, I denied it was happening to myself at first but soon knew that this was only a false hope.

OH MY GOD, DOES THIS MEAN I'M OLD NOW?

Panic

After denial there is usually panic. All the societal implications of baldness start running through the sufferer's head. To be bald you are older, boring, unmanly or unwomanly, possibly diseased, and deficient in sex appeal. There are no positive characteristics associated with baldness. The fact that more victims in our society do not go into a severe state of depression from hair loss is a great demonstration of the resiliency of the human species. But panic can cause its own set of problems.

I have seen countless patients who, in the rush to stop or cure their hair loss, cause worse damage by either using deleterious chemical hair treatments, or by getting their heads shaved by some slick outfit which then attaches some hairpiece or system prematurely to their scalps. As mentioned earlier, this causes traction baldness and furthers psychological damage.

I had one patient who, in the panic of hair loss, proposed to a girl he really didn't love because he felt getting married would relieve his worries about hair loss decreasing his sexual appeal. The girl finally figured out the scenario and brought him in for a consultation. He underwent, successfully, a hair transplant and now they are good friends, but not lovers.

ARE YOU LOOKING AT ME? THEN WHO ARE YOU LOOKING AT?

Anger

You wash your hair every day and you're very careful about blow-drying, brushing, or otherwise damaging it—you haven't done anything wrong. So someone else, the victim at this stage reasons, must be to blame.

I have had fathers (with both full and bare heads of hair) come into my office with their balding offspring and spend thirty minutes discussing with me how it's not their fault. "Tell him it's not my fault," they'll say. Some then add reflectively, "Maybe it's his mother's." Similarly I've seen children point to their parents and quite loudly blame them as well.

I have seen patients get so angry after being "ripped off" by useless cures that they have even assaulted the people who sold them the snake oils when they couldn't get their money refunded.

The angry hair loss victim is a volatile one. I had one mother the other week call and tell me that she would do anything to help her nineteen-year-old son with his thinning hair. She further told me he was assaulting his kid sister when she would comment on his problem and he even hit the mother once when she broached the subject.

This is real anger, and as such, needs to be dealt with.

No matter how angry you get, remember one thing—it's the fault of genetics in most cases and pointing blame does not cure the problem. Although you know you want to do something about it (or you wouldn't be angry) you will still suffer through phase three in some form before you can proceed to phase four.

WILL I EVER GET ANOTHER DATE?

Withdrawal and Depression

Depression often does occur at the onset of hair loss and in some cases never goes away. The image we see in the mirror can certainly affect our conduct in society.

Someone has made a comment! Now you wear hats and avoid photographs. You avoid social situations because they may lead to embarrassment (remember my wig story). So it's time to hibernate. You find reasons not to go to the beach or swim or play in active sports where you can't wear a hat. Sometimes you just stay home. I had a female patient who was so traumatized by her hair loss that she wouldn't attend her daughter's wedding. I have also seen young men who have dropped out of school to avoid potential embarrassment. Many times their mother or father will bring them to my office and describe their antisocial behavior. The children will blame their parents for causing this condition as if their parents had a choice. Often times even their posture will change. Young men will slump and look sullen so they can avoid eye contact with the outside world. I, myself, would constantly make excuses to avoid any situation that could expose my hair loss.

In other words, you are letting your hair rule—and maybe ruin—your life.

It has become more common for me to see patients on antidepressants while they are giving me their medical histories. When I ask them why they are taking medication, their answer is invariably the same, hair loss. Some try therapy to combat the problem, others have reverted to drinking alcohol and or drugs to anesthetize their minds. But all have one aspect in common. They are depressed about their hair loss.

One patient spoke with me for an hour about his concerns. Henry N. was single and went to a country and western night club to meet a date. He was dancing with a girl he liked when another man came up and asked the girl to dance. He said, "Excuse me, she's with me," and the answer directed to the female was, "Why do you want to dance with this baldie?" He then pulled the patient's combed-over hair upward, revealing his bald area and sending Henry running. Henry came to see me after his depression became so bad he actually considered suicide. His mother came with him to the office after voicing her concerns about his psychological situation. He's now undergoing a transplant. Henry acted probably at the point he was entering the next phase, acceptance and resolution. His resolution, though, could have been tragic.

ACTUALLY, DON'T YOU THINK IT LOOKS A BIT SEXY?

Acceptance and Resolution

Next comes acceptance. Many men simply accept hair loss as part of the passage of life. After all, hair loss is a normal genetic trait passed on from generation to generation. There are certainly many handsome masculine individuals who have chosen to accept or simply ignore their hair loss. This is certainly the best and healthiest attitude one can take. Whether we are destined to be short or tall, handsome or homely, athletic or awkward, hairy or bald, these are all part of the genetic cards we are dealt and we should accept them.

Some men go so far as to embrace baldness. They wear it as a badge of honor, proudly proclaiming I am Bald and Proud. The Bald-Headed Men's Club of America, in Moorehead, N.C. has members from around the world who correspond and get together to support hair loss as a mature, sexy, virile appearance that society should look upon with admiration. Most men deal with hair loss as inevitable and natural and move on with their lives and careers. Appearance is comprised of many aspects, not the least of which is our personality and intelligence. A good personality and interesting mind have more of an influence on our attractiveness than any physical characteristic.

Unfortunately not all men are created entirely equal and

acceptance of the inevitable is a characteristic that varies dramatically from person to person. Hair loss is not something we are born with; it happens later in life, after we have gotten used to seeing ourselves a certain way. Our hairline is the frame of our face, and just as an attractive frame and matting compliments a picture, our hair compliments the features on our face. As with a picture, if we take away the frame, the face appears more ordinary and far less attractive.

The feeling that their appearance has suffered is a significant reason why men often do not accept baldness. For every actor, model, or politician I have seen for consultation about hair loss, I have seen hundreds of very normal men who typically are not very vain or concerned about their appearance in general, but cannot accept going bald. Age also is not a factor. Although generally a young man suffers when going bald more than a mature male in his fifties or sixties, I often meet with older men who feel their hair loss has unfairly aged them. They do not want to change their appearance but rather want to restore it to a fairer picture of who they are.

When consulting with patients I am always first concerned with their motivation. If a young man is looking to restore his hair so he can feel better about himself and has a reasonable expection of the result I can achieve, then he is a good candidate for hair restoration surgery. If on the other hand the prospective patient feels that having hair will make him more popular and desirable to the opposite sex, or that his hair will help him succeed in business and life, I will discourage this person from undergoing permanent hair restoration surgery and rather encourage counseling and a more temporary hair replacement solution.

Just as hair loss is not the cause for all your problems, it is also not the cure. For individuals to succeed socially and professionally it is much more important to have personality, intelligence, and strong character than a fuller hairline. Hair can improve our appearance and self-image but only strong character and motivation can help us to succeed in life. It is important that when we look into the mirror for answers to our problems we should look deeper than the surface for the solutions.

You now know it's true and it's time to either accept it or do something about it.

- You can shave your head as many sports figures do
- You can begin to look into various treatments

But first you do what most of my patients and I have done.

You consult your hairstylist.

THREE

WHAT CAN MY HAIRSTYLIST DO? "THE ILLUSION OF HAIR"

Your hair has thinned. You may either have a bald spot or simply "see through" hair. In any case, it's time for that first consultation with the person who you feel knows you best; for most people, it's their hairstylist.

WHAT HAIR STYLES CAN HIDE HAIR LOSS?

Lots of people have thinning hair. It's how they style it that can make a difference. In my practice, for those patients just suffering from very early hair loss, I will often send them to a good hairstylist as well as make recommendations for treatment of the problem.

A good hairstylist knows how to cut and shape thinning hair to help maximize its covering power. Privacy is important and I often tell people to ask for your hairstyling consultation "behind closed doors" (neighbors in the salon and barber shop love to listen to other's problems). Your professional may recommend a "body wave" to thicken limp or fine thinning hair, or he/she might layer it to give the look of significant thickness. The hairstylist may also cut portions of the thinning areas shorter because *short*, not long hair, covers better. This is because the weight of longer strands of hair tend to cause it to separate. Thinning hair becomes less noticeable when the hair is shorter because it is acceptable to see some scalp through shorter hair (think of military recruits who even with full heads of hair exhibit a thinning appearance after the short haircuts given in basic training). Combine this with slightly longer hair elsewhere and a lower part, and you've effectively camouflaged the problem.

Hair color helps as well. When hair is thinning, the less the contrast in color between the hair and scalp, the less noticeable the problem. Thus blond-haired Caucasians look less bald than their dark-haired counterparts with the same degree and pattern of hair loss.

WHAT SHOULD I NOT DO?

- Don't braid or use rollers to give your hair extra body—they will cause breakage and further thinning.
- Don't try to dye your hair because the chemicals (as mentioned) can permanently damage the scalp.
- Don't keep your hair too long because the weight of long hair tends to make it separate and thereby expose thinning areas of the scalp.
- Don't blow-dry your hair constantly and too closely with hot air as this will also cause hair breakage.
- Don't brush your hair constantly because this too will cause breakage and thus thinning of your hair.

WHAT HAIR CARE PRODUCTS HELP CONCEAL HAIR LOSS?

Hair care products can often help your assault on thinning hair. Your hairstylist can help you choose those that are best suited for you.

Shampoo

Shampoos advertise all sorts of claims. According to the professionals I consulted, these are the most important things to remember.

1. Change your shampoo regularly; the hair adapts to the same product if used daily. The goal of shampooing is to leave the hair clean and manageable.
2. Try to use a hydrophilic (or water absorbing) shampoo which helps swell the hair shafts and makes hair appear thicker.
3. Beware of "coating" shampoos which in actuality coat your hair with a chemical and so make it appear dirty and less manageable.
4. A detergent shampoo is meant to cleanse the scalp by removing sebum (the discharge from sebaceous glands) and dirt; however, some sebum is necessary to retain your hair's sheen.
5. Foaming shampoos are not better than nonfoaming ones.
6. Kinky hair should be shampooed less often than straight hair as sebum is necessary for grooming kinky hair.

Conditioners

Conditioners counteract the detergent effect of shampoos. They "smooth" the hair shaft and remove static cling while attracting light reflection. Thus, they create shiny, manageable hair.

Remember, different hair types (e.g. fine vs. coarse hair) adapt differently to different agents. Coating conditioners (hair thickeners) can actually add such weight to fine hair as to make it unmanageable. This is why your stylist is your best guide to hair care products.

Gels and Mousse

In the professional hair care world, gels and mousse are known as "left in" conditioning agents. They can vary from the pomades that African-Americans often apply to kinky hair to add luster and body, to the moisture-absorbing "gels" that add thickness and body to limp hair. Many of these products also contain silicone which helps the hair feel smooth and silky to the touch.

The primary purpose of these products in our context, though, is to give more holding power to thinner hair.

Hair Spray

Hair spray, like mousse and gels, is directed at giving increasing holding power to finer or thinner hair. The base of many hair sprays, however, is alcohol and can thus dry and dull hair. The key is to be smart and sparing. Hair should be able to blow somewhat freely in a breeze. The helmet look may be okay to some, but can be as artificial as a bad hairpiece to many others. Hairstylists have the proper training in what is best for you.

Perms and Waves

Perms and waves are chemical methods to make fine, thin, or straight hair appear thicker by making it wavier or curlier. They generally will last about four months and can be helpful to those people in various stages of hair loss. They can also be damaging, as I have mentioned before. If you are uncertain if a perm or wave will help, consider asking for a *water wrap,* which simulates the perm without the chemicals. If you like it, finish the perm, if not, save yourself four months of bad hair days. If you decide to go ahead, make sure you go to a professional who performs these techniques regularly and will carefully monitor the application.

Haircolor

As mentioned earlier, many people do not realize that what makes thinning hair very obvious is the contrast of skin and hair color. For example, thinning black hair on a fair-skinned person is much more obvious than the same amount of blond hair thinning on the same skin type. Therefore, proper hair coloring (vs. skin) and highlighting can help hide a "multitude of thinning sins."

When I gave hydrogen peroxide as part of the post hair transplant cleansing routine, I often got Caucasian patients telling me that their hair looked better already. What they did not realize was that their new blond highlights helped downplay their thinning problem.

Once again—all chemical treatments of hair can be dangerous and should be performed only by a competent professional.

FOUR

WHICH NONSURGICAL TREATMENTS FOR HAIR LOSS DON'T WORK?

Well, here you are—if you're reading this chapter you may have decided to do something about your hair loss. So let's explore your options for nonsurgical treatments and hopefully you will avoid the pitfalls most hair loss sufferers encounter.

It's really amazing when I see all of the intelligent people who come to me and describe some "crazy" treatment they have tried. I remember at least six people who entered a study which prescribed rubbing female cow urine twice a day into their scalps. (They didn't grow hair but I bet they got a seat on the subway.) Similarly there was someone ten or fifteen years ago that had many men and women walking about all day massaging their scalps to increase circulation and grow back their hair. They did as well as the cow urine group.

The stories go on and they aren't just from the latter twentieth century.

HOW TRUTHFUL ARE ADS FOR MIRACLE CURES?

Let's consider an ad from 1905 in a prominent magazine published in New York: "A Scientific Method of Growing Hair." The ad depicts a balding man wearing on his head a large vacuum cap similiar in appearance to the old beauty parlor hairdryers. It covers most of his scalp.

The text explains: "It is a known fact that blood conveys nourishment to all parts of the body. It is likewise known that exercise makes the blood circulate, and where there is no circulation, there is no nourishment."

The advertisement goes on to say that "the lack of proper circulation of blood in the scalp due mainly to congestion produced by artificial causes starves the hair roots and produces falling hair (baldness)."

The Evans Vacuum Cap purports to provide scalp exercise which draws rich circulating blood to the scalp and will thus nourish the shrunken hair roots, causing them to regrow.

The advertisement further states that the cap is easy and pleasant to use, requiring only three to four minutes of wearing daily. It then gives a method for you to test it by using it for two to three minutes and then checking your scalp to see if it has a healthy glow (today, we'd call it irritation). No glow, then you are not a candidate for this treatment. Of course, everyone is a candidate.

Finally, the ad offers you a money back guarantee from a bank in St. Louis that you must contact yourself if you are not satisfied. (Not easy to do in 1905.)

Sounds pretty familiar and convincing, doesn't it?

Let's analyze this ad and see what made it so successful.

1. It makes sense that the hair will not grow without blood supply—a claim we still see today—*it is not true.*

2. The device makes sense in its claim to replenish blood supply, a claim also playing on logic but absolutely *not fact.*
3. The scientific test—sounds good.
4. *The money back guarantee*—This is the single *best* selling claim for these charletons. They count on normal reasoning, if the product doesn't work, how could the company refund your money and still stay in business?

   Well statistics show that only 5 percent of dissatisfied people ever request a refund. It's a cheap price to pay to convince you to try the product. And try the product many will do. In other words, a money back guarantee implies warranteed success and adds to the product's credibility. Fortunately for these people, the lack of refunds makes the guarantee an inexpensive selling ploy.

If the above sounds familiar, it's because this ad could appear in the 1990's and still be successful. That's because we all want to believe there's an easy way to cure the hair loss problem—and thus we accept the ads as gospel, even in today's more skeptical climate.

Ads proclaiming cures for baldness still flood both the print and entertainment media. I constantly receive mail order catalogs (I probably made the list by ordering from one of them) that pitch products that treat or "cure" hair loss. What I find most interesting is that many of the active ingredients were discovered in some faraway location, such as Tibet or the valleys of Hungary, so their effectiveness is impossible for us to verify easily. One of my favorite cures was based on the research of a professor from the University of Helsinki, Finland. It seems he accidentally discovered a cure for baldness while conducting cancer research.

Although the cancer treatment was nonprescription and not FDA approved, the company who marketed the cure claimed it was safe and effective and made it available via mail order. Ten years and hundreds of millions of consumer dollars later, the firm has been found guilty of false advertising in the Ninth Circuit Court in California. The company president was held personally responsible because he "acted with reckless indifference to the truth," according to the judge's decision.

It took the Food and Drug Administration ten years of hearings to ban the over-the-counter sale of products claiming to cure baldness, but in 1989 they finally did. So how do the scams continue?

One way they go on is as a result of manufacturers claiming their products don't cure hair loss, but instead cleanse the clogged pores that trap your growing hair so to allow the hair to escape from under your scalp and reappear. It sounds dumb, but untold numbers of people (including a friend) tried these expensive products anyway.

There are many other hair restoration cures that are more myth than medicine. Just glancing through tabloid publications and catalogues constantly reveal new ones appearing almost monthly. Always ask your hair loss professional before trying them.

CAN ACUPUNCTURE RESTORE MY HAIR?

Acupuncture may be helpful in curing some minor ailments, and has been used successfully to prevent pain during even major surgery in China, but it can't solve every problem. Hair loss is not caused by nerve damage or impairment and, therefore, nerve stimulation through acupuncture will not help cure it. Fortunately acupuncture is rarely touted today (as it was three decades ago) as a treatment for hair loss of any cause. If you see an advertisement for this please do two things: send me a copy and then forget about it.

I HAVE HEARD ABOUT RARE RUSSIAN HERBS THAT SUPPOSEDLY CURE BALDNESS. DO THEY WORK?

No. These miracles of modern fraud were first brought to my attention by a Russian herbologist, who came to see me at my office. She and her bald husband touted the effects of this miracle drug with which she claimed to have extensive experience in the Soviet Union. She left Russia because of political oppression, but fortunately escaped with this secret ingredient and the "recipe" to make the formula. I asked her why her husband was bald and her answer was simply, "It doesn't bother him."

I next asked to test the formula but she was fearful that I would steal the secret from her to profit for myself. I suggested that she conduct the test herself and that I examine and document the results. She agreed, made the first appointment, and never showed up again.

Forget Russian herbs, rare or not.

CAN MASSAGING MY SCALP FACILITATE HAIR GROWTH?

In 1981 Autumn Press published *Growing New Hair*, a book which touted the profound effects of scalp massage.

The premise was that the hair roots were dying from lack of proper circulation. Only massage could return the proper blood supply to them and with it would come hair regrowth. This idea was logical and very appealing to most people, and in a simple way it almost made sense. The problem, in my opinion, is that scalp massage doesn't make sound medical treatment sense in curing baldness.

In 1983 I debated the author on "New England Today," a regional New England News program based in Boston, Massachusetts. My question to her was, if a lack of circulation caused the hair to fall out on the top of the scalp, then why would transplanted hair grow in this same "infertile" region? After some careful thought, she replied that transplants "damaged the scar tissue." That answer made no sense to me, but the question certainly does. I would love to see good clinical studies on her part to substantiate the theory. To date, I've seen none.

I used to tell patients who asked about the massage treatment to improve circulation that if they wanted to know how good the blood supply to their scalp was to prick it with a pin. (*Do not try this at home or elsewhere please!*) The point is that the scalp has the best blood supply of any region of the body and massaging it is like throwing a cup of water into Niagara Falls and looking for the splash.

WHAT VITAMINS PROMOTE HAIR GROWTH?

Although vitamins are important and can affect hair sheen, lack of them is not a cause of hair loss.

You should not confuse hair quality and hair care with hair loss. Vitamins and minerals may be partially contributing to good hair care, as well as other vital body functions, but they will not cure hereditary baldness. The person who sold Vitamins For Your Hair along with Right Places Breast Enlargement Pills served prison time for mail fraud. There is a good reason for this.

Spend your money on products that help, not ripoffs. If you take vitamins they should be for the right reason, not for some false hope.

IF SCALP MASSAGE WON'T WORK, WILL ELECTRICAL STIMULATION OF THE SCALP?

A few years back, I helped explore a New York treatment with a consumer reporter, Rosanne Coletti of CBS News. She went to the doctor performing it and questioned him with regard to its validity. He presented her with an old paper from a little-known journal claiming that this process worked well. Remember, journal articles are printed but not checked except in the most prestigious of publications. So the doctor offered no quality scientific substantiations for the treatment, just a six-to seven-thousand-dollar tab for trying it. The doctor who was performing this, furthermore, was not licensed in New York state according to CBS's research.

The basis for this treatment probably goes back to the early 1950's when studies showed that topical irritants (like peroxide) could cause dying hairs to be stimulated to regrow about 1⁄100 of an inch. The effect doesn't last but this led to the claim, *it grows hair.* Yes, I guess it grows hair 1⁄100 of an inch, but this will certainly not make your day. Stay away from this treatment until some better proof comes along. I always welcome new good research data in evaluating or reevaluating any opinion of treatment validity that I express.

ARE THERE ANY CHEMICAL SCALP TREATMENTS THAT WORK?

For almost forty years, two companies existed that performed scalp treatments with special formulas to regrow your hair. Their claims changed over time to encompass the idea, "HOW DO YOU KNOW IT'S HEREDITARY HAIR LOSS?" The doubt that this created was designed to compel you to try these expensive weekly treatments just in case the cause of your hair loss was not hereditary.

Well, one clinic closed after a sex scandal among workers, and the other just faded away along with its false hopes and people's hard-earned money.

The theory here is the same as that behind electrical stimulation, an irritant causing a minuscule amount of hair growth. The formulas always contained hydrogen peroxide to make the scalp tingle and thereby convince the user that it was working. I'm glad at present (who knows for the future) that this treatment is just a memory.

HOW IS THE GOVERNMENT TRYING TO PUT A STOP TO THESE SCAMS?

The number of false cures will inevitably get larger. When asked, the Food and Drug Administration will tell you that enforcement is a real problem.

The U.S. Postal Service began a campaign in recent years trying to stop the fraud as well.

An ad placed by the U.S. Postal Inspection Service points out probably why most vendors will not use the U.S. mail to send you their remedies. The postal service is a government agency and therefore has federal regulations that private carriers do not. A reliable vendor will not hesitate to use any carrier including the U.S. mail. Others may be afraid of mail fraud. Nongovernmental carriers such as U.P.S. or Federal Express therefore become convenient safe seconds.

FIVE

WHAT ARE THE ACCEPTED NONSURGICAL TREATMENTS FOR HAIR LOSS?

WHAT IS ROGAINE™ (MINOXIDIL) AND HOW WAS IT DISCOVERED?

The following is paraphrased from the "History of Minoxidil" by Gerald R. Zins, Ph.D., of the Upjohn Company, published in the *Clinics of Dermatology*, Oct.–Dec. 1988.

Back in the early 1960's, Upjohn began testing a compound it had first ordered out of an American Cyanamid chemical catalog. The initial tests were to decrease stomach acidity but researchers soon learned that it was more valuable as an agent to decrease high blood pressure. The side-effects of water retention plus heart and lung damage were soon clear, but by 1971 it was a sought-after oral drug used in lowering dangerously high blood pressure when other safer medications failed.

The medicine was administered to patients under strict monitoring. It soon became clear that patients on the medicine for longer than two weeks had an interesting side-effect, hair growth. This was further explored after a patient whose severe high blood pressure (and who happened to be bald) was treated with minoxidil by mouth. After several weeks the bald spot disappeared. Dermatologists tested the drug topically on upper arm sites with a similar hair growth result. Safety concerns held back further testing because of the dangers of oral minoxidil.

Dr. H. Irving Katz reviewed the efficiency (effectiveness) of topical minoxidil as safe and that it does stimulate new cosmetic hair growth. He felt, however, that for most patients, "The restorative effect lacks a great cosmetic impact." He went on to say, "In most patients, the results are subtle and consist of barely perceptible new vellus hairs; however in some patients these vellus hairs become pigmented, thicker, and longer and can be classified as nonvellus. Patience on the part of the patient and physicians is required."

Dr. Katz reviewed the results from thousands of patients and over 315 dermatologists. The article in the *Clinics of Dermatology*, Vol. 6, No. 4, Oct.–Dec. 1988, goes on to provide additional information I believe to be true today.

"Subjective perception of dense coverage occurs in less than 5 percent of the patients, whereas approximately 20 percent experience at least some minimal nonvellus hair coverage. Our group and others have noted retardation of hair loss or actual decrease in the diameter of the bald area in patients using topical minoxidil, which implies a stabilization and modifying effect. In general, younger patients (less than forty years) with a smaller balding diameter (less than 10cm) on the vertex and having at least 100 terminal or intermediate hairs (2cm or longer) in a one-inch balding area seem to respond more favorably. Frontal hairline alopecia does not seem to respond as well as vertex alopecia, although there are few relevant objective studies.

"Hair growth has been maintained for years with topical minoxidil use; however, twice-daily applications seem to be necessary for the best effect. Regrettably, if topical minoxidil is discontinued, increased hair loss and further progression of baldness occurs within two or three months. Therefore, use of topical minoxidil in androgenetic alopecia requires a long-term commitment, most likely for the duration of an individual's life.

"The efficacy of a drug such as topical minoxidil cannot alone be measured by raw data on objective or subjective static observations. The ultimate reputation of the drug, and potentially the prescriber, will depend on the realistic expectations of the patient. Efficacy has different meanings to the FDA, statisticians, physicians, patients, spouses, and pharmaceutical companies. Depending upon the criteria used, the efficacy of a medication for androgenetic alopecia in a real sense depends upon 'the eye of the beholder.' Slight restoration and prevention of further progression of baldness may be extremely relevant to an individual who is balding. To the casual outside observer, however, little overt efficacy may be appreciated.

"The high restorative expectations of an individual patient must be tempered by the stark reality that probably less than 5 percent of men with androgenetic alopecia achieve significant cosmetic improvement. Most of the remainder of those who respond will demonstrate some increase in nonvellus hairs, but not significantly enough to have an overt cosmetic impact."

Time has shown us that we rarely see great hair regrowth with Rogaine. It seems to work best when slowing down or stopping hair loss in young people just beginning to lose their hair. The product (called Regaine outside the U.S.) has also been reported by many to work for a limited time only in many patients and has not lived up to its expectations.

I have used Rogaine (minoxidil) in my practice for over

fourteen years and I am still waiting for dramatic regrowth results. Hair loss stabilization and its use in hair transplantation (see later chapter) offer me more hope. It also has been reported to work well in some of the other hair loss causes such as alopecia areata. The other problem is it's a lifetime commitment at thirty dollars per month and patients tell me that for the result it is just not worth it.

On April 15, 1996 Rogaine became available without a prescription in the United States. The advantage, over the long term, will hopefully be lower costs and easier compliance for patients using this medicine. Unfortunately, the patient loses the professional guidance of a skilled physician who can objectively evaluate whether the medicine is working or the patient is simply wasting his time and money.

WILL ROGAINE HELP WOMEN?

Where I and many of my colleagues have seen better results using Rogaine is in treating female hair loss. I first used it on my wife, who had thinning in the front of her scalp after taking Accutane. She stopped the Accutane and I gave her a six-month trial of Rogaine which worked quite well. Her hair loss had disappeared. I then took her off of the Rogaine and six months later the problem reoccurred. I gave her another six-month trial and now, six years later, the problem has never reoccurred. I've seen similar results with hundreds of my female patients and my colleagues report similar results. Upjohn, in its studies reported in "A Woman's Guide to Understanding and Treating Hair Loss" published by them, reported that "Rogaine was significantly more effective than placebo [similar solution without minoxidil—the active ingredient in Rogaine] in regrowing nonvellus hair in women with androgenetic alopecia (female baldness).''

Effectiveness was measured by patient and physician evaluation and by nonvellus hair counts. Between 19 percent and 25 percent of the women using Rogaine for thirty-two weeks felt that they had achieved at least moderate hair regrowth, compared with between 7 percent and 12 percent who used a placebo (a similar solution without minoxidil—the active ingredient in Rogaine).

Almost two out of every three women in the Rogaine group were evaluated by physicians to have regrown some hair: 13 percent had moderate regrowth and 50 percent had minimal regrowth. The rest (37 percent) had no regrowth. Thirty-nine percent of the women in the placebo group were evaluated by physicians to have regrown some hair.

However, when the actual number of newly regrown hairs in the 1 cm^2 area of the test were counted after eight months of treatment, the group using Rogaine averaged more than twice as much regrowth (22.7 more hairs) as the placebo group (eleven more hairs).

I have empirically tried Rogaine on some women just after delivery (never during pregnancy) with good results. Their history was hair loss in their sisters and mothers after child delivery and they sought anything to prevent themselves from becoming the next victim. I can't give you a scientific basis for it, but it seemed to work.

Thus the treatment of female hair loss is one of the true strengths of this drug. It promotes hair regrowth. Since then I have used Rogaine on over two hundred women with close to a 40 percent rate of hair regrowth of all degrees. I still use it for this today.

HOW DOES MINOXIDIL WORK?

According to Dr. Vera Price, clinical professor of Dermatology at the University of California in San Francisco, "Rogaine works in part by partially enlarging miniaturized follicles and reversing the miniaturization process. This prolongs the growth phase of the hair cycle, allowing the hair to become longer and thicker. And with more follicles in the growth phase at the same time, it is possible to see improved coverage of the scalp.

"Although the growth phase may be prolonged, the follicle will continue to cycle. Several cycles may be necessary before maximum potential hair regrowth can be achieved."

HOW EFFECTIVE IS RETIN A?

This medicine, introduced for the treatment of acne and surface facial wrinkles, has shown some side effects of hair growth. No large study has sustained these results. We do know however that retinoids (a derivative of Vitamin A) are necessary in women for the sustained growth and color of hairs. It is for this reason that Retin A has been tried and applied to both men and women suffering from hair loss.

IS RETIN A MORE EFFECTIVE WHEN ADDED TO MINOXIDIL?

Back in 1984, Dr. Vera Price reported that the combination of minoxidil and Retin A works better especially in the front of the scalp. None of my colleagues nor myself have found this to be true, although I wish it were. What it seems to do is potentiate the effects of minoxidil alone in slowing down or stopping hair loss in the early patient. In one study in Japan, they felt that when in combination, the Retin A helps the absorption and thus intensified any positive effects of even a more dilute suspension of minoxidil. Here a 1 percent suspension could act as if it were really 5 percent. Side-effects were rare.

WILL MINOXIDIL WORK BETTER WHEN COMBINED WITH OTHER SUBSTANCES?

No matter what you read, I wouldn't advise you to use minoxidil in combination with any miracle cure. Any result you obtain—give the minoxidil the credit and save the cost of the hype ingredients.

DOES A 5% CONCENTRATION OF MINOXIDIL WORK BETTER THAN THE 2% CONCENTRATION FOUND IN ROGAINE?

Clinical trials just haven't proven this to be a great improvement over the current 2 percent suspension. Five percent minoxidil is not FDA approved as of this writing.

BECAUSE TESTOSTERONE PLAYS A LARGE ROLE IN HAIR LOSS, WILL PROSCAR, A DRUG AFFECTING TESTOSTERONE LEVELS, HELP CURE HAIR LOSS?

Merck and Co. has FDA approval to use Proscar (the trade name for finasteride) to shrink the prostate in older men, thus allowing them to avoid prostate surgery. It probably works by altering testosterone levels in men by blocking its conversion to dihydrotestosterone, which as we have seen, is a major culprit in hair loss. It is a pill, and has been reported to decrease male sex drive and possibly cause male breast enlargement. I am not ready to try it yet until I learn more about the possible side-effects to the body. Often it takes years to learn what the long-term consequences of an oral medication are. I would rather wait and see the longer-term studies. (For further information, please see the chapter on future treatments near the end of this book.)

WILL CORTISONE AND PROGESTERONE INJECTIONS PREVENT HAIR LOSS?

For years people thought that we could give progesterone and/or cortisone injections directly into the scalp to stop 5DHT from reaching hair follicles and destroying them. They are however, expensive, painful, and only minimally effective in male and female pattern baldness. We will discuss their possible future role later in the book.

IF A DECLINE IN ESTROGEN LEVELS CAUSES HAIR LOSS IN WOMEN, WILL REPLACING THE ESTROGEN BRING THE HAIR BACK?

One thought was that if loss of estrogen in women would cause hair loss, replacing it might stop it. Studies now show that outside estrogens do not work the same as the person's own production of this hormone and therefore don't prevent hair loss. Therefore postmenopausal or postsurgical younger women who have suffered a decline in estrogen production and, therefore, a resulting decrease in estrogen levels cannot use replacement therapy to save them from female pattern hair loss. The earlier studies which showed topical estrogens in slowing down or reversing early hair loss have not been substantiated to date. One wonders if an extract of one's own estrogen used topically could treat female baldness. There are no studies to date.

SIX

HOW CAN I COVER MY HAIR LOSS? FROM HAIRPIECES TO SYSTEMS

Caesar used olive branches and bangs to cover his balding pate. Others imported lighter color hair from the Nordic regions or Northern Europe to create their "upper class" hairpieces. Powdered wigs were the rage of the elite throughout Europe from the fifteenth through the mid-nineteenth century. Kings and queens, and those in the English court system even today still wear wigs. Throughout the twentieth century, the hairpiece or toupee has still been an important cosmetic solution for baldness or thinning hair for men and women from movie stars to blue-collar workers.

Today, the product may still be a hairpiece, but I doubt you'll find very many people who will call it that. Today's hairpiece is light years ahead of what was available even ten years ago. New technologies have helped the hair replacement field develop "hair systems" that are amazingly light and natural. To help understand where the technology is today, we need to first go back and understand the ancestor of today's hairpiece.

WHAT IS A HAIRPIECE?

A hairpiece is a covering made of anything resembling hair. As I mentioned above, many items were used throughout history as a "covering" for a balding scalp. In fact, it is known that wigs were made of everything from sheep's wool to goat hair, and even cotton or synthetic fibers are included.

The base of hairpieces in the past were usually a heavy netting in order to provide durability. Much lighter nylon mesh hairpieces were made but primarily for actors and actresses in motion pictures where their lifespan was generally brief. They would easily tear or lose the attached hair, but they looked very natural in front of the camera. The hairpieces were applied with glue and makeup was patted over the front silk mesh, hiding it from the camera. The mesh was also very fine so there was no bulkiness that needed to be disguised.

The traditional way wigs were attached required them to have a stronger base. Double-stick (two-sided sticky) tape was cut and applied to various portions of the base of the "piece" and then attached to the scalp by pressure. This double-stick tape was similar to carpet tape and, thus, wigs were nicknamed rugs. The wig hair would then be combed to blend into one's surrounding natural hair and, in general, hair spray would be applied to help fix the piece into position.

One of my favorite stories involves a husband and wife who came to see me about hair transplants to correct the husband's hair loss problem. The husband was concerned and was asking questions, but five minutes later his wife suddenly began yelling at him. She said he looked fine the way he was and that he was "stupid" to change what God had given him. I asked the wife if she wore makeup (believe me, she did) and why. Her answer was, "It covers my acne scars." I then asked if God gave you a certain look, isn't it stupid to change it. Her answer was "Mind your own business" and so I did. Two years later the husband came for his transplant, his wife having had a rhinoplasty (nose job) and blepharoplasty (eyelid job) in the recent past. She no longer objected and instead stated, "I want him to look like a father and not a grandfather when our four-year-old grows up." She told me she would give her permission for his procedure if I had a way of covering his thinning hair during the procedure so it wouldn't be an embarrassment to *her*. We got him a temporary partial hairpiece. The procedure was a success. (His wife has since had a facelift.)

WHAT ARE THE PROBLEMS ASSOCIATED WITH THESE HAIRPIECES?

These pieces were easily detected for several reasons.

1. The hairlines were often too abrupt and thick and, therefore, appeared unnatural.
2. The natural part never looked natural.
3. They generally had too much hair, making the wig look obvious and the wearer look silly.
4. Perspiration would loosen the double-stick tape and a good brisk wind could lift the hairpiece up at the worst possible time.
5. Wind could blow the attached hair into unnatural configurations.
6. When submerged in water, as when the wearer

was swimming, the hairpiece could become dislodged easily.

7. In the past, the hair color would rapidly oxide (fade and discolor) especially in sunlight, so soon the wearer had "two-tone" hair. The improvement of synthetic fibers over human hair have made more current systems more rigged and less likely to fade, however.
8. Most importantly, most wearers had to apply the piece themselves daily and would often miss a spot which should be covered. They also might easily place the wig too low on the forehead or even slightly sideways because of the poor vantage point they inevitably had when applying the hairpiece. I once had a patient that had come in for a consultation and was so nervous showing me his balding area that he reapplied the hairpiece backwards before leaving the office. Fortunately my staff pointed out this mistake to him. He later returned for a transplant and when he took his hairpiece off I noticed that he now had the words "front" and "rear" embroidered into the base of his hairpiece. After a successful transplant result, the patient was able to still utilize his old hairpiece for another family member. Front and rear direction was not as important here.

WHAT IS A HAIR WEAVE?

Because of the problems with hairpieces, the hair replacement firms of the 1970's introduced a new process—the hair weave.

Hair weaving involves the creation of wefts (braids) of one's remaining hair along the sides and back of the head. This was intertwined with thick thread in order to facilitate the attachment process. The hairpiece base was then "sewn" to the wefts of hair to secure it to the scalp.

WHAT PROBLEMS ARE ASSOCIATED WITH A HAIR WEAVE?

The immediate problem with this process was that the weaves tended to be large and bulky because the hairpiece had to overlap the existing hair in order to hide the braid. Also, the front (the most obvious aspect) of the hairpiece still needed two-sided tape to attach it since there was nothing to braid the front to.

Soon it became obvious that there were other problems.

1. Because the weave was attached to your existing hair, it required frequent rebraiding and reattachment as your surrounding hair grew (usually every four weeks). This required the wearer to go monthly for "maintenance" to the seller and thus endure a constant expense.
2. Recoloring was required every three months and soon it became necessary to buy additional hairpieces to help prolong the life of each weave unit. The additional hairpiece also provided a backup for the other hairpiece when it was in for prolonged service. This too became expensive.
3. After approximately six months of constant wearing, users began to develop traction baldness in

> the attached braided areas (see Chapter 1) and these soon became permanent areas of hair loss.

I often saw, in my practice, patients who would come in with circular areas of shiny baldness along with normal male pattern hair loss. They looked like they had alopecia areata (see Chapter 1) but it was soon obvious that these abnormal circular bald patches developed in the spots where their hairpieces were braided. People with extensive braiding would often develop an artificially created widening of their hair loss problem and would continuously need larger and larger pieces for coverage.

One of the biggest problems I noticed among long-term wearers of weaves was the result of their inability to keep their scalps clean. Patients would tell me that when they would ask the maker of their hairpieces how to clean their scalps, they were routinely told to buy a Water-Pik™ and stick the tip under the continuously loosening weave. It was not uncommon for me to find fungal or bacterial infections on the scalps of long-term wearers of weaves, and I would often have to treat them with antibiotics and antiseptic scrubs before attempting to perform a hair transplant on them.

Often times in my practice men would come in, their hairweaves, which they had cut off, in hand, complaining about the constant maintenance costs, discomfort, and scalp irritation. Immediately after attachment, patients would describe the headaches and uncomfortable feeling of their hair being constantly pulled. This would especially be prevalent during sleep when they would wake up every time they turned in bed. The ones who tolerated this would soon find the circular bald patches I described above.

Eventually the makers of hair weaves changed their marketing strategies, and many young consumers with early hair loss began buying hair weaves believing that their own hair would be woven through the weave. ''Integrated'' was the marketing term. These people would leave the hair replacement center soon to discover that their existing hair on top was trimmed or shaved and the hairpiece was simply tied to whatever surrounding hair they had. This often ''married'' the user to the piece because of fear of embarrassment upon its removal. Later modifications involved weaving snaps onto one's remaining hair at the fringes allowing the hairpiece to be easily removed. (See insert photo 1.)

WHAT ARE THE BENEFITS OF A HAIR WEAVE?

Despite the downsides of hair weaves, for many men who opted only for a hairpiece, the hair weave offered a new level of security and piece of mind in social situations. Finally they had hair that was windproof and wouldn't shift during physical contact. And if properly and frequently maintained, weaves offered significantly better freedom and appearance than a traditional toupee.

WHAT IS BONDING?

Technology has improved the attachment process considerably in recent years, and bonding has become the trend of the nineties. Basically, in bonding, a hairpiece is glued rather than tied to the scalp. The process was first tried in the late 70's and was known as fusion. The agents used for the bonding however have remained similar. They are dif-

PROS AND CONS OF SYNTHETIC FIBERS AND HUMAN HAIRS

Synthetic Fiber		Human Hair	
PROS	**CONS**	**PROS**	**CONS**
1. Color does not fade	1. Does not reflect sun	1. Color can be blended with ease	1. Can be heavy weight
2. Does not lose curl patterns	2. The ends may freeze up when exposed to heat (sun, swimming pool and sauna)	2. Hair has movement (when style is at least 10" or longer)	2. Can shed faster
3. Lightweight	3. Hard to blend the color of the unit with client's own hair	3. Can be cared for as client's own hair	3. Can be rather expensive
4. Available in much greater variety of colors	4. Tangling problem when hair is longer than 10 inches	4. Great flexibility in styling (when weaved in)	4. Not too much variety in stock (especially in long hair units)
5. Less shedding	5. Color cannot be changed	5. Great flexibility in coloring	
6. Greater variety of styles in stock	6. The proper degree of heat cannot be used to style ethnic hair	6. Undetectable	
7. Less costly	7. Does not absorb stray oil	7. Is not afraid of heat (natural sun, curling irons, blow drying, etc.)	
		8. Can be worn in a swimming pool or Jacuzzi	
		9. Can be re-texturized when needed	
		10. Responds well to home maintenance products	

Source: American Hair Loss Council

ferent forms of cyanoacrylics otherwise known as quick-drying glue. The old bulkier pieces didn't take well to this process, but new lighter ones with bases made of plastic and light meshes seem ideal.

WHAT ARE THE ADVANTAGES OF BONDING?

1. Since the system doesn't require attachment to surrounding hair, the size of the piece can be customized to the size of the bald area instead of being bulky and oversized to cover the braids.
2. These systems have a more natural appearance especially when a person's existing hair can be combed in. (If you remember Ted Danson on "Cheers," he wore a system to cover a bald spot in the crown and then combed his existing hair back onto it.)
3. It does not lift as the person's surrounding hair grows because it is not attached to the surrounding hair.

Bonding thus involves the attachment of anything from a tiny patch of hair to fill in a small bald spot in the crown, to a full hairpiece to cover a large bald area. It has to be reattached every three to six weeks with a form of Krazy Glue™ applied directly to the client's scalp. The purchase of two systems is usually necessary since the unit will still require regular maintenance for coloring or replacing lost hair.

Most units still use human hair because the synthetics, although more durable, lose any wave or curl when wet and will not regain that wave or curl when dry. Instead, the wearer must have the unit reserviced.

WHAT PROBLEMS ARE ASSOCIATED WITH BONDING?

As with its predecessors, bonding has its pitfalls as well.

1. The glue can loosen in the front especially when the skin is oily or sweaty, causing it to lift up.
2. Many patients of mine have had the uncomfortable feeling of always wearing a hat.
3. When participating in sports or when exercising, the wearer's own hair will wet and flatten with sweat while the unit hair remains unchanged, thus making the difference in the two hairs more obvious.
4. One's natural hairline and part recreation is still detectable in many cases.
5. Most importantly, in cases where there was still a lot of the person's own hair on the top of the scalp, the glue process will cause the same damaging hair loss effect as traction alopecia, resulting in permanent additional hair loss.

Although I don't see the many clients who are probably happy with the bonding process, I have literally seen thousands who are not. I had one grown man actually crying in my office when, the day after the process, he woke up to find the unit half off and his head shaven underneath. We converted his unit to berets for temporary anchoring and successfully performed a hair transplant on him.

I have seen other patients who have told me they were informed that their own hair would be pulled through the system. Instead they found themselves with a shaved glued head. And when I worked as a consultant on a story for the consumer reporter on WCBS T.V. in New York, others interviewed by Rosanne Coletti said they never understood that what they were getting was a hairpiece attached with glue.

The Department of Consumer Affairs of the City of New York has cited several of these bonding establishments for false advertising. This helps point to a major problem which has arisen in this field—*ethics*.

WHAT SCAMS ARE ASSOCIATED WITH THE BONDING PROCESS?

Patients often tell me they never would have bought a bonded system if they knew what it was. Unfortunately, there is little or no regulation in the field and ripoffs are all too common.

Yet there are decent professionals who provide a service here. Ads taken out by some establishments begin with the headline "Don't be scammed," but people still are—they want to believe there's an easy way to "cure baldness."

One giant scam that I helped stop involved an outfit in New Jersey that advertised a permanent solution for baldness. In their national advertisements, International Cosmetic Labs (ICL) claimed that their process, which took a day, would attach as much hair as a person wished and this would last "forever." Tens of thousands of balding people fell for this and wound up with a wig sewn dangerously into their scalps for a ridiculous sum of money. Due to undercover operations with CBS News, the story about ICL was exposed and soon they were out of business with a giant class action suit filed for fraud against them.

The horror here is that what these people did caused scarring, pain, and infection to patients as well as destroyed their hopes and finances. As a result of the ICL scandal, laws have been passed in New Jersey and New York outlawing this procedure.

In my practice, I have performed hundreds of corrective procedures on these victims. Unfortunately, when the patients come to me for help, they have already been disfigured and must have something done to help them. Fortunately, hair transplantation has solved the problem for many of them. Sometimes the scars are so low on the forehead, however, that some will remain visible.

WHAT ARE SKIN GRAFTS FOR HAIR, AND WHAT DANGERS ARE ASSOCIATED WITH THEM?

In another scam conducted in the early eighties, ads stating "Skin grafts for hair" made hopeful patients think that they were receiving the most modern medical procedure to restore their hair. The pictures looked great.

But what did they receive?

The patient would go to the doctor's office where he would be sedated. Then skin from his groin was taken and placed on the scalp forming three loops of skin on top of the head. Next, a hairpiece with three attached plastic strips was given to the patient. All he had to do now was slide the plastic strips under his three disfiguring loops and presto—skin grafts for hair.

Of course the victim never knew this would occur. He also learned the hard way that with sports activities or if someone tugged on the piece, the loops of skin could tear, causing bleeding and pain and worst of all, cause the piece to fall off. In addition, the price he was quoted did not cover the surgical cost of creating the loops, thus making the final cost prohibitive.

It was a pleasure helping to close U.S. operations of Look International, the company responsible, and a challenge to reconstruct the damaged scalps of over two hundred patients I treated with this problem. I was successful in removing the loops with scalp reductions and then going on to transplant the patient's own hair.

WHAT IS HAIR INTEGRATION?

One process which is the legitimate method of adding hair without shaving or bonding a hairpiece is hair integration. In this process, various amounts of hair are attached to a weblike cap. Then, by using a tail comb, one's own hair is drawn through the webs and blended with the existing hair. It adds thickness, length, and body. The hair is synthetic and color matched. Because it is not a hairpiece, it rarely inhibits physical activities. This, as all hair replacement, does require frequent maintenance but is the best addition I've seen for those (especially women) who have thinning hair with no clear bald spot.

HOW DO YOU FIND A REPUTABLE HAIRPIECE DEALER?

One way is to contact the American Hair Loss Council in Chicago, Illinois (Consumer Hotline 1-800-274-8717). This nonprofit organization tries to police this vast field and has help organize a credentialing committee to oversee what's right and wrong in hair replacement. They publish consumer reports on all aspects of hair replacement written by experts in the field and are available to help guide the unwary person away from disappointment. Their quarterly *Hair Loss Journal* covers every process and aspect of hair loss and its replacement, and reprints are readily available by calling the hotline number.

The second way is to read and review the advertisements in your local papers, magazines, television commercials/ infomercials, and telephone directories. Third would be to consult a friend, colleague, or family member that has had a relationship with a hair replacement professional.

Once you have collected the names of centers near you, call and prequalify the center. Ask them if they have the knowledge, the products, and the abilities to fulfill all of your realistic expectations. Request any printed information that may be available to you. Once you have received this information and studied everything you should, choose several centers, schedule an appointment to personally interview the center's professionals and to see the operations of the center and the center's product lines. Ask for client referrals and, if possible, ask if you can speak with a client of the center or meet with him/her in person. Discuss pricing for not only the addition but also the ongoing services. Choosing the hair replacement center is extremely important. It should be as important as the addition itself. The center should be neat, organized, professional, helpful, ready to provide support service, support products, and have a comprehensive knowledge of your needs and how to achieve your goal.

Once you have completed and made your choice, it is time to set the appointment for your design and fitting. Make sure that the staff is completely aware of your desires as well as your concerns. Establishing everything during this consultation will help both you and your chosen professional, and will prevent you from being disappointed with the hair addition once you receive it.

Remember one word, *experience.* There are many inexperienced people in the field and that even if they use the best product, they are not experienced enough to properly fit the client. Interview several. A rapport with the dealer is nice, but ask to meet and talk to several clients. Also check if he keeps old and new clients separated (either by appointment or separate waiting rooms). Sit in the waiting room and talk to those with you. Don't be shy, you may be sorry later.

Also check with the Better Business Bureau locally. Anyone can have one or two complaints, but beware of a large volume of them.

Remember, this is a commitment. Take your time and choose wisely. Do not be misled by slick claims and unrealistic promises.

HOW DO I JUDGE HAIRPIECE QUALITY?

In choosing a hair addition you should make sure that the addition is designed to meet your expectations in lifestyle and look. The addition should be made of suitable materials for your chosen method of attachment, your lifestyle, and desired look to insure that you receive the optimum life expectancy and minimum disappointment out of the addition. In order to avoid problems in the future the method of attachment should be determined during the design phase. The type of hair should be chosen according to your predetermined realistic expectations in your image, your lifestyle, and method of attachment.

Human hair is best suited to an individual that is expecting to continue a more active lifestyle and more flexibility in styling. Synthetic hair is best suited for an individual that does not require as much versatility of styling and a somewhat less active lifestyle. If a guy is a construction worker or hard in general on his hair system, the foundation should be thicker and stronger. If the unit has a lace front and thin foundation, it will never last. A good hairpiece for one person may be the wrong and thus a bad hairpiece for another. Also, how the person will wear his hair will help determine the type of hair and foundation that should be used. For example, synthetic hair is not useful for someone who wants to keep his hair permed because if it gets wet, the perm will permanently disappear.

The best way to judge the quality of the hairpiece is to rub the hair between your fingers. If it feels real with smooth texture, if it brushes well and has body, if it looks like healthy hair and is not dry or worn out, then it is more than likely a good quality unit.

WHAT IS THE DIFFERENCE BETWEEN A GOOD ADDITION AND A BAD ADDITION?

This is a question asked time and time again and has a simple answer. A good hair addition is the one that lives up to your expectations and desires. That is why it is so important to choose a hair replacement professional that will work with you to develop not only a good hair addition but also a long standing relationship of quality services and products for years to come.

CAN MY GIRLFRIEND/BOYFRIEND RUN THEIR FINGERS THROUGH MY HAIR?

Yes. The development of finer materials and better methods of maintaining the hair/fibers gives you a more natural feel to the entire addition. Materials for the addition are constantly being researched to create a finer/thinner almost invisible look. The texture, color, and consistency of the hair are carefully blended together, giving you hair that feels as good as the hair that once grew out of your head. The synthetic fibers have been refined to their finest level giving it an almost exact match with human hair.

Always keep in mind that without the proper care and maintenance by you and your chosen hair replacement professional your addition will not live up to what you expect out of it. You must develop a commitment to a routine maintenance program in order for your new hair to continue looking, feeling and acting like your own.

CAN I CONTINUE ACTIVITIES SUCH AS SWIMMING WITH MY ADDITION?

It depends. If the addition is designed from the beginning with this in mind you should not have any problems with maintaining a physically active lifestyle. That is why it is very important for you to choose the right person and facility to develop, design, and maintain your hair addition.

The wearer must keep in mind that, after activities such as swimming, they must blot the addition dry after coming out of the water. Do not rub with a towel. This will help maintain the quality of your addition and prevent or minimize damage to the unit.

WHAT SHOULD MY ADDITION COST?

Hair additions range from as little as four hundred dollars to over three thousand dollars. The average cost of a quality hair addition is approximately $1600. The question, however, should not be, how much does the hair addition cost, but what is it worth to you?

Custom pieces are priced between $850 and $3500. The higher prices are generally seen at "chain centers" who advertise heavily while the lower prices are usually found at small shops. The right price for a good custom unit should be $1200 to $1500. The monthly maintenance including cleaning, adding hair, and coloring should run seventy-five to ninety dollars per month for all services on the average. Those interested in coloring should make sure the color added is by powder dye. This is because it is gentle on the hair. Commercial color dyes such as Clairol are much harsher and can damage the system's hair, thereby shortening its life.

In addition, having two units is far better than one because servicing will be more timely and the client will be less likely to abuse the unit before he finally repairs it.

Ready-made hairpieces (which cost from five to six hundred dollars) can be 95 percent as good a fit and quality as the custom piece and might be good for those on a budget, or those just not feeling the need for custom work. It doesn't hurt to try a ready-to-wear piece before investing in the more expensive variety. Remember, you can purchase two or three ready-to-wear pieces for the price of a single one. You may consider purchasing one custom-made piece and one ready to wear as a backup. In this case, you can compare both pieces during actual use and see if the off-the-shelf variety will work for you.

Specific products are also made available for home care as well.

Keep in mind that a less expensive hair addition may not live up to your expectations and that the most expensive may not live up to its claims. I again stress that you should make your choice intelligently, basing it on facts and not on emotion and hype. Be aware of the person that sells too hard, for he may have very little to offer.

CAN I HAVE AN ALLERGIC REACTION TO MY HAIRPIECE?

As for allergic reactions, hypoallergenic double-stick tape is rapidly replacing the older stock and so are new glues.

Experts have told me that because of these changes reactions to the bonding agents are becoming rarer. I have seen several severe skin reactions (with a generalized rash and redness over the whole site of the attachment, requiring topical steroids and in one case oral antibiotics as well). The same experts also tell me that synthetic hair rarely causes a rash. They have collectively seen only two reactions (rash only) in the past thirty years which disappeared when human hair was substituted in the unit.

WHAT ARE COSMETIC COVERUPS?

By now most of us have seen either the infomercial or the spoof of it about spray-on hair. Although you may find this product and other cosmetic coverups amusing, they can work for the right patient.

Recently, I had an eighty-year-old lady come with her daughter to the office for a consultation for a hair transplant. She said she has lived the last twenty years with a bald spot just behind her hairline (she claimed it was hereditary in her family and had a dermatologist's evaluation confirming it). She had heard transplants had come a long way and had met one of my patients who recommended seeing me. She was on blood thinners and I didn't feel it was safe to transplant her, so I did the next best thing. I sprinkled some Great Coverup "Artificial Hair Powder" onto the bald spot and presto—spot gone. I keep samples of this product in my office for patients as a cosmetic coverage aid during hair transplants. She was so thrilled that she asked if she could call the toll-free ordering line from my office. I obliged and felt good knowing I made this senior citizen very happy. It was a far nicer way to solve a problem than to just tell her she's not a candidate for a transplant.

Her daughter even baked cookies for the office.

For many people, cosmetic coverups are temporary camouflage during hair replacement surgery. But for others, they can supplement a poor to fair result from prior procedures as well as help those who are not candidates for other surgical procedures because of health reasons to achieve their desired results. They are also excellent for those people looking for a simple way to thicken the appearance of thinning hair.

Remember, camouflage is not for everyone. I remember one infomercial where a man who was totally bald on the top of his head "sprayed" hair on. He looked like he had just fallen into a vat of tar. *You must have some hair in the area you wish to use the product for it to work!!!*

WHAT ARE THE BEST COSMETIC COVERUPS AVAILABLE? WHAT ARE THE BENEFITS AND PITFALLS OF EACH?

1. Temporary hairpieces. As I mentioned before, these are great aides. They can be made to clip to existing hair for security and to prevent damaging adherence to fresh surgical sites.
2. Invisible concealer. This is inexpensive makeup with a fine applicator which works great on the scalp reduction lines as well as on small areas of scabbing. Most are hypoallergenic and I have never seen a topical reaction to it. Clearasil works great, too!
3. DermMatch. This is a water-resistant scalp coloring which can be safely applied over even fresh surgical sites to give the appearance of thicker hair. It can also be used in *sites with existing thin hair as well.* It does not run when wet nor when caught in the rain and it looks very natural. The problem is applying it. You must use your finger-

tip for good application, although every package now comes with a new applicator to remedy this. It also can stain your fingers if not washed off immediately, requiring longer, harder scrubbing to completely remove the coloring.

4. Couvré. This is an excellent scalp colorant (as per DermMatch) and applies very easily. The problem with this product is that it runs in water (which can be embarrassing) and stains your pillowcase and shirt collar. The company has notified me that the newer product is more water resistant. Used correctly, it can be a big help because of the quick application and excellent coloring matches.
5. Super Million Hair. This Japanese product works great on very fresh surgical sites as well as in thinning hair. It is a fiber that adheres to surrounding hair to give it increased fullness and thickness. It sprinkles on easily and does not run. Like all colorants, It is available in a variety of shades and colors.

   Super Million Hair is no longer available in the U.S. The Japanese version unfortunately contains some non-FDA approved ingredients and I have seen two cases of scalp inflammation after use by women who had no prior transplant surgery.
6. Great Coverup. Because I found Super Million Hair so helpful, I was thrilled to see a similar product released that was made in the U.S. and whose ingredients were all FDA approved. I called for samples and had my staff try it (we are always the guinea pigs). The result, a great product in five colors and lousy packaging. Don't let the package or the silly name fool you—this works well for easily and safely covering thinning spots. We saw

no adverse reaction in the group of twenty of us who tried this for two weeks (previous reactions were within seventy-two hours). Although I would advise any patient to be careful and consult their physician before using any product, this physician loves the DermMatch (especially for the hairline) and the "Great Coverup" best for general camouflage. (See insert photos 2–3.)

7. Spray-On (shoe polish). I left this for last because this is where it belongs. The spray-ons can be messy and can also stain pillowcases and clothing. More importantly, in many cases they inflame the scalp and in my opinion are not safe for use on recent scalp surgical sites.

   My experience, with all these products is extensive, having performed over thirty thousand procedures in twenty years. The above information is the consensus of many patients. I have no financial interest in any camouflage products, only the personal interest I have always had in my patient's well-being.

My Advice: Take all the legitimate aides and help you can get.

WHERE CAN I BUY THESE PRODUCTS?

Almost all can be purchased either by mail order or in some cases are available in larger drugstore chains. Below is a list of how to get more information on each product and/or ordering them.

Invisible Concealer	Available at all drugstore cosmetic counters.
DermMatch	9812 Falls Road, Suite 114–22; Potomac, MD 20854. 1-800-826-2824.
Couvré	Spencer Forrest, Inc.; 3 Sylvan Road S.; Westport, CT 06880. 1-203-454-2733.
Super Million Hair	No longer available in United States. However, the Great American Coverup fills this need safely and effectively.
Great Coverup	More Hair Cosmetics, New York. 1-800-874-HAIR
Spray-Ons	Mail-order catalogue and/or major drugstore chains in the hair care department.

SEVEN

WHAT IS A HAIR TRANSPLANT?

WHAT IS THE HISTORY OF HAIR TRANSPLANTS?

The idea for transplanting hair to cure baldness is over 150 years old. In the first published treatise in 1822, J. F. Diefferbach discussed his investigations in transplanting skin, as well as feathers and hair. His first clinical trial was indeed successful with all three materials.

In the early part of this century, papers began appearing in the medical literature discussing grafting to cover defects caused by injury. As early as 1911, an article by J. S. Davis was published entitled "Scalping Accidents." The study was conducted at John Hopkins Hospital. But the true first utilization of hair transplantation to cover cosmetic hair loss must be credited to the Japanese. Dr. S. Okuda, in the late 1930's, began experiments in transplanting small grafts of hair roots in Japanese women in order to create and thicken eyebrows. He devised and introduced the circular punch (which is similar to a cookie cutter) as a device that could be sharpened and make a clean cut in the scalp thereby not damaging the hair follicles beneath the skin's surface. He went on to describe how by placing these circular grafts of skin, hairs, and roots into receptor sites (the bald area) that were a bit smaller in diameter, his result was thicker and cosmetically superior. The result was not perfect and looked a bit clumpy upon close inspection, but women were excited to have growing eyebrows once again.

Unfortunately, World War II disrupted his work, and many of his reports on his progress were lost.

Based on much of the research of skin grafting which demonstrated that the graft always behaves as if it were in its original position, Dr. Norman Orentreich went to work developing the modern theory behind today's hair replacement surgery. What Dr. Orentreich did was transplant grafts from both normal and bald sites to areas on the scalp that were both hairy and bald. What he found confirmed that if the donor site contained healthy hair and roots, no matter where it was transplanted on the same patient, it would grow hair. Transplants of bald skin would not grow hair even if transplanted to areas on the scalp of normal hair growth. (This helps explain why many of the "cures" we talked about earlier in the book are nothing but scams.) The original hair transplants were performed in the mid 1950's and several years of followups showed continuing growth of hair in the recipient areas, even with the first patients still continuing to bald. Dr. Orentreich developed the modern-day circular punch used in hair transplantation and its exclusive use lasted for another two to three decades.

I entered the field in 1975. At that time, we were taught by the few physicians performing hair transplantation that the circular grafts from the back (the plugs) should be spaced apart for healing and compressed into smaller receptor sites for increased thickness of growth. The term plug came about when people described placing a larger circular graft into the smaller site by pushing it in, similar to recorking a wine bottle.

Well back in 1975 we grew hair! It was thick and for

1975 looked good unless you wanted to comb it back and reveal the hairline. Traditionally we left space between the plugs creating the term "cornrow" or "Barbie doll look" and it took careful and creative combing of hair to help cover these problems. Yet we grew hair and that was what many balding men were seeking.

At the same time the concept of strip grafting was introduced by Dr. Charles Vallis. Here, the first attempts at transplanting a relatively large strip of hairs from the back of the scalp in order to achieve better cosmetic effect and density took shape. The problems here were that although the skin would "take," there wasn't enough blood circulation to allow the follicles to survive. Large strip grafting disappeared very quickly. Flaps were also introduced in 1975 by Dr. Juri of Argentina. These will be discussed in another chapter.

In the late 1980's, although we were growing substantial amounts of hair, we needed to refine the hairlines. In my case, I began studying many men and women, my partner included, with good God-given natural heads of hair. What I noticed almost universally was that nobody's hairline goes from "desert to forest" no matter how thick the rest of the hair is. So, although other physicians had described using smaller grafts on the hairline, I still sought a better way to improve the results. (I also had a vested interest in this as although the wind could no longer blow off a hairpiece on me now that I was transplanted, it could certainly reveal my cornrow hairline.) Smaller grafts looked better, but they still were not "better enough." I had a local instrument company make very small circular punches and decided to try reversing the hair direction on the hairline to create a feathering zone. I was the guinea pig.

This worked so well that I began to routinely incorporate this practice for all my hair transplant patients. I called this procedure blend grafting and for me, the age of refinement of results was upon us.

Back in the late 70's and early 80's, I routinely had both dermatology and plastic surgery residents coming weekly to my office to observe the hair transplant procedure. These interactions proved helpful in obtaining new ideas for improving the procedure as well as in training some well-educated doctors in my techniques, which many carried on and made their own contributions to the field. Soon one of my students, now a practicing dermatologist at Cornell–N.Y. Hospital, and I began research in hair loss as well as its corrections. We were both former baldies and our interest was both personal as well as professional. In 1986 we published a paper on seven methods of improving the hair transplant result in the *Journal of Dermatologic Surgery and Oncology* (12:7 July 1986). Our subsequent innovations were chosen for the 1988 yearbook of plastic and reconstructive surgery.

What was state of the art in 1980's, however, was passé by the 1990's, so it was time to go back to the drawing board. People's expectations were changing, and undetectability, as well as hair growth, became our goal.

The first big attempt at improving the transplant came with the notion that more hair was not better. It was time to decrease the size of the plug in order to avoid the big "tufts" of hair. Doctors now started reversing themselves and began transplanting larger numbers of smaller grafts. Dr. Emanuel Marritt reintroduced the concept of single hair transplants for hairlines and most doctors scrambled to learn the technique. Big plugs were cut in half or even quarters to make them smaller, but unfortunately the long-term result was a head of smaller tufts that was not at all thick.

Then, in the early 1990's, some doctors experimented

with transplanting increasing numbers of one or two hair grafts. The idea was to create the illusion of hair without the look of a transplant. Well, it doesn't look like a transplant, but unfortunately it still looks like the patient needs one, even after long sessions and huge expense.

With HMOs and insurance reimbursements to doctors in all fields causing panic among physicians, the field of hair transplantation became increasingly attractive. No longer would I see the same small group of us at meetings discussing our ideas and results. Instead, I witnessed hundreds of doctors in all fields coming to weekend seminars and then going out to practice hair transplantation. The idea of performing one to two hair grafts only was attractive because the physicians were taught that it took considerable experience to use larger grafts successfully and by avoiding them, they could avoid problems. Schools popped up at expensive prices to train the doctors in hair replacement procedures. Diplomas were issued after as little as two to three weeks of training.

Now, in the late 90's, hair transplants have joined the hair replacement industry as a business. It disgusts me, and I hope what I write here will help guide you around the pitfalls.

Please remember: There is no substitute for quality, education, and experience.

WHAT IS A HAIR TRANSPLANT?

A hair transplant is a minor surgical procedure where healthy areas of skin, hair, and their roots are transplanted from the sides or back of the head (the donor area) to bald or balding areas of the scalp of the *same person* (the recipient area). Transplanted hair will generally continue to grow permanently because it is taken from an area where the hair roots were never programmed to fall out. The hair transplant graft (transplanted section) always retains the same characteristics as where it comes from, thus the hair will continue to grow at the same rate with the same color and characteristics as it did prior to the procedure. It will even turn gray as you age.

In the past the areas from which the hair had been taken were allowed to remain open and heal naturally, creating a pegboard effect in the donor area. Today's donor areas are sutured closed and heal with thin scars in most cases.

Donor areas are chosen to match as best as possible the type of hair that should grow in the area being transplanted. For example, hairline hair is generally taken from lower on the back of the head or the lower sides where the hair is finer and will help feather the front.

HOW IS A HAIR TRANSPLANT PERFORMED?

When you arrive for a procedure, you should expect the following series of steps. First the area to be treated should be reviewed with the *physician*. If a new hairline is to be created, you and the physician *should* discuss the best design for your appearance and style. Often I have patients come in with pictures of themselves taken in second grade. Here they have a kid's hairline which may look good in public school, but will certainly not be flattering as an adult. Believe me, I've seen the wrong hairline many times and it can be a disaster. My common remark to all new patients is to err on the side of conservative. It's easy to lower a hairline, but almost impossible to raise one. If they insist,

I next show them a picture of Eddie Munster and ask them if this will make them happy. If it does, I send them home with a stern warning.

Once the hairline is established, you should expect 35mm photos to be taken so the extent of hair loss can clearly be documented for later review. Often I find patients coming back to the office not realizing how bald they used to be. This is because the hair growth occurs over time and it's easy to forget from whence you came.

Next you should expect the donor area to be selected and your hair above pinned up to cover it immediately after the procedure. Both the donor and bald areas are then cleansed with an antiseptic solution. Local anesthetics are next administered with or without premedication or nitrous oxide (laughing gas) to numb both areas.

In my office I give the laughing gas while numbing and then use a long-acting local anesthetic (Marcaine) to help prevent a wear-off ache hours later. As a patient myself I can tell you this really works.

You should never expect your head to be shaved. Recipient sites are then cut and prepared in the balding area (the types vary as we will discuss later) according to your predetermined pattern, for hair replacement result. These sites are replaced by the healthy donor grafts positioned at an angle to duplicate your hair's natural growth pattern.

The procedure can take anywhere from an hour to over twelve hours depending on who's doing it and the type of the procedure you're having. My typical procedures take two hours (most patients are restless when it's much longer) and the patients watch television or videotapes during it.

At the end of the procedure, you may or may not have a bandage applied for overnight. This varies with the doctor and type of procedure. Both are acceptable practices. The bandages, however, are much smaller than the old days.

We no longer put giant turbans on the head post-op. I once had a patient back in the 70's who went from his transplant procedure to a theater in the city playing a popular science fiction alien movie. He stood outside the theater and signed autographs as people were exiting thinking he was in the show. Other patients would put big fake rubies on the front of the bandage turning it into something funny rather than scary for their families. All of this is part of transplant history now.

DOES IT HURT?

Now this is the $64,000 question.

The answer is—it depends on your doctor's technique and skill in numbing along with your own tolerance for any pain.

What I have found most effective in my patients is to prenumb the recipient and donor areas with a very small amount of dilute local anesthetic. This feels simply like a mosquito bite (without the dreaded buzzing). Next I give the patient laughing gas. I then administer the regular local anesthesia into the prenumbed area and find that most patients feel virtually nothing.

Once numb, you will hear funny noises (the scalp conducts sound) but will feel no pain.

Long-acting anesthesia really helps to prevent the wear-off ache and makes the transplant very comfortable at night.

Other doctors perform nerve blocks to the nerves supplying feeling to the front and back of the scalp. These shots are given in each eyebrow, and although safe, do not have great appeal to a patient who is awake. Some doctors will premedicate patients with Valium or the like before the procedure, although this makes driving home impossible if you are alone. General anesthesia, although it sounds appealing, can be quite dangerous and is therefore not indicated or necessary for basic hair replacement surgery. The after-effects of general anesthesia can be nausea, vomiting, headaches, etc; in other words, a post-transplant nightmare. Most doctors stick with what works best for them.

WHEN WILL THE HAIR GROW?

All scalp hair grows in a growing phase (anagen) and in a resting phase (telogen). Every hair on our heads replaces itself every six years. Think of the resting phase as a three-month hibernation cycle where the follicle is alive under the skin but there is no cosmetic hair produced. After its three-month dormancy, the follicle once again produces a new cosmetic hair.

Certain factors will throw growing hair prematurely into a resting phase. Any type of minor trauma, such as surgery, will fool the follicle into an early three-month resting cycle. This is no different than moving a flowering plant from one soil area to another. The plant roots survive, but the flower may not.

Transplanting hair temporarily interrupts blood supply and thus will cause the growing hair to shed. As such it's not unusual for patients to call frantically telling me that the transplant didn't work because the hair fell out. In fact, the hair only *temporarily* falls out and the root remains in a three-month resting phase. The new hair then begins to grow and will resume its old genetically programmed cycle.

And no, they don't all fall out every six years.

Occasionally, patients will come in to the office telling

me that some transplanted hairs continued to grow and never did fall out. Instead of the patients being excited that they are ahead of the game, they instead want to know why the rest of the hair isn't continuing to grow as well. What this shows is that often the smaller (or narrower) transplant grafts will grow quicker because they heal faster. But this is only thin frontal hair and the patient should assume then the best is yet to come. So to answer the question directly—new hair growth will start in two to four months in general. For some reason it starts quicker in the front than in the back (crown), and the more transplant sessions you have, the longer it takes for the subsequent transplanted hair to begin growing.

WILL ANYTHING SPEED UP THE GROWTH?

A few years ago, a New York dermatologist published a paper comparing the speed of hair growth after transplant with and without the accompanying use of minoxidil. He felt it helped in healing and thus earlier hair growth. Unfortunately, he based his claim on only twelve patients. I went to the drawing board and did the same trials on over two hundred patients. The result—in some cases, the hair never fell out, in others it made no difference, but in no cases did it hurt. As such, I dip all transplant grafts in minoxidil (with patient permission). I also place my patients, if they are willing, on minoxidil for three months after. My feeling is that minoxidil is a vasodilator (it opens blood vessels) and as such speeds fresh blood supply and healing to the new hair grafts.

WHAT IS HAIR TRANSPLANT SHOCK?

Very often I have patients come into the office with very little hair loss in an area. They tell me it bothers them while I'm trying to figure out why. Well if the hair is just beginning to thin and I perform a transplant in the hope of thickening it, I may be causing transplant shock. This is a condition where the surrounding hair goes into the same resting stage as the new transplanted grafts. As a result, the person looks balder after the procedure. The hair, in general, will grow back although both patient and physician will probably talk often during this period.

WHAT IS BLEND GRAFTING?

Blend grafting is a technique that was developed to eliminate the hard or "cornstalk" look of the hairline. It entails the use of various size grafts (down to a single hair) which help feather the hairline to achieve a natural look. Your doctor should be able to position micro and single-hair grafts in a staggered placement of the newly created hairline to create an impressive, aesthetically appealing result. As I stated, I was the "guinea pig" of this idea, and once an idea works on me with my coarse dark hair (better than having a shiny bald scalp) I then apply it to my patients. Blend grafting is a technique that is not easy for the amateur transplant doctor, and if your doctor doesn't believe in it, maybe you should check on his or her experience in the field.

WHAT TYPES OF HAIR TRANSPLANTS ARE THERE?

Let me answer this question by telling you that a transplant is a transplant—in other words all hair transplants involve moving hair from an area of healthy growth to a bald area. But this is where the similarities end. So let me categorize the different types of hair transplant procedures.

WHAT IS A PLUG?

A plug is a circular hair transplant graft taken from a donor area (usually made by using a power tool) and transplanted to a prepared circular site on the top of the balding scalp.

As I described earlier, it's called a plug because a slightly larger graft is "plugged" into a smaller bald site, which can cause a thick, tufted result. Since the plugs are slightly separated from one another, the result was the often-described cornrow effect. Different size circular "plugs" were inserted between the prior healed or growing ones, but there was always a small space between the grafts making them noticeable, especially in dark-haired patients with contrasting light-colored skin.

Recently, I had a patient come in to correct an old pluggy transplant. He told me he was a police officer and had finally got tired of being called plug head by those he arrested. Nobody likes an Achilles heel.

Generally plugs were very large in diameter and would contain fifteen to twenty hairs. The typical procedure would require three or four visits of about one hundred plugs each in a very bald (class V) gentleman. (See Norwood's diagram, page 7.)

Hair was usually styled to the side to cover the hairline and any of the plugs in the center of the bald area which were always spaced further apart than those on the hairline or frontal region. We used to tell most patients, "Look it's not perfect, but at least you have hair."

There were two schools of thought in the past. Some doctors believed that only twenty to thirty plugs should be transplanted in each (of multiple) sessions. Others felt that larger sessions were better for the patient and the result because circulation, and therefore, subsequent growth lessened with multiple procedures.

WHAT IS A MINIGRAFT AND A MICROGRAFT?

After seeing the result of large plugs only, doctors began to integrate smaller circular grafts between the previous cornstalks in order to soften the look. Dr. L. Lee Bosley, in the 70's, trademarked the names minigraft and micrograft. Others (myself included) began calling these microsized and minisized plugs at about the same time all in effort to be able to describe what we transplanted on patients in a standard way. By using smaller plugs (three to five hairs = minigraft) the result was softer, but we were still making a critical error in judgment. Our plugs were still one half mm wider than the site we put them into. This discrepancy therefore became more pronounced in the smaller plug that was transplanted. Also, round small plugs still were not the perfect answer for the hairline.

The micrograft (one to three hairs) was our first true attempt at single hair transplanting and helped considerably in creating a hairline that looks natural.

WHAT ARE SLIT GRAFT TRANSPLANTS?

Slit grafts were the first real attempt at avoiding the plug look. In essence, they were simple cuts made in the bald area into which we inserted small strips of hairs and their roots. The problem, of course, is that no bald tissue is removed and thus, like trying to lay too much carpet in a room, you will eventually get buckling (or in some cases pitting) to accommodate the extra tissue. This is called the *carpet effect*. When a person has only thinning hair (as in female pattern hair loss) slit grafts can be useful because they add hair without removing the surrounding thinner hair. But let me emphasize that if an area is balding significantly, slit grafts can look worse than the old plugs because they can look like little tufts of hair coming from beneath the surface of the scalp.

WHAT ARE LASER TRANSPLANTS?

Laser transplants are cuts made in the top of the scalp in an attempt to eliminate both the tufting look of plugs and slits. A high-energy "ultrapulse" (meaning short bursts of cutting light) carbon dioxide laser is employed to make the sites on the top of the head. These laser cuts are really slots and not slits because lasers cut by vaporizing a small thin strip of tissue. Into these small slots (decompressed slits) the same strips of hair and roots are placed, and the result is remarkably natural growth. The problems are as follows.

1. Laser grafts only have been successful growing one to three hairs each, so density is a problem.

2. Not all the grafts take. You can lose up to 30 percent of the transplanted hair.
3. Its almost impossible to precisely densify the previous laser slits without destroying some prior transplanted roots.
4. Lasers clot blood flow and some blood flow is necessary to nourish the new grafts.
5. Positioning of the hair in natural growth angles is quite difficult.

Even with all these problems, the progress in the concept of transplanting without plugs is leading the way to even newer ideas in creating a natural-looking result.

WHAT ARE SINGLE-HAIR TRANSPLANTS AND MEGASESSIONS?

Single-hair transplanting is the attempt to once again avoid "plugs" and thereby create a natural result. In this procedure, large numbers of single-hair grafts, sometimes even several thousand, are made from strips of hair removed from one's donor area, and are individually inserted into the top of the scalp. These megasessions can take up to twelve hours each. The benefit of this type of session is that the result looks natural, but as several patients have asked me, "Where's the hair?"

Megasessions can only create a thin result, and often, the patient is fooled into believing that one giant session will solve his whole problem. I had a patient and his wife, recently, who after three megasessions and about $30,000 came to see me. Both agreed that although the result didn't look like he had had a transplant, he still looked like he needed one. Two sessions of larger denser grafts helped solve this problem. (See insert photos 4–5.)

WHAT ARE LINEAR GRAFT HAIR TRANSPLANTS?

After carefully observing the results of all the different types of hair transplants mentioned above, I began working on building a better mousetrap. These were the parameters that had to be dealt with.

- The round plug gave density but looked "pluggy."
- The single-hair graft was natural but thin.
- The slit graft was the right shape but tufty.
- The laser slit graft was a small slot that, though natural, was still thin and inconsistent.

In 1993, I began experimenting with altering the shape of the transplant punch (the device we use to make the recipient sites) in order to simulate the laser result of natural growth, but to have the advantage of varying size and direction of grafts. Making the tool was not as difficult as sharpening it, and my first attempts at making a successful device left me with shoulder damage from trying to cut with a knife blade that was not razor sharp.

Because I worked with ex-military and military reserve medical personnel who now reentered civilian life, I had access to a resource group with tremendous talent. Some had engineering as well as combat medic training, and could offer me technical assistance I needed to develop my product. Of particular help was Walter Lozano (USMC) whose technical skills made my dream a reality.

Walter worked for months on creating a narrow punch

that was so sharp that if you dropped it on your foot, it could cut through your shoe. He helped me develop sixteen different length punches which could transplant a single up to twelve hairs in a linear fashion. By this, I mean that the hairs were behind each other in a strip that was only ½ to 1 mm or ¹⁄₅₀th of an inch wide. These grafts healed better and quicker than laser grafts, but more importantly also afforded me the ability to vary direction, shape, size, and distance between the grafts. They healed like small cuts (plugs healed like gashes) and grew as natural appearing as megasessions (except we now achieved density as well). No longer would one have to sit for twelve hours in a procedure just to achieve a see-through look.

We next developed a tool to create a "perfect fit" for the grafts we made to fill the slots. This new group of patented technology is rapidly improving patient speed, comfort, and result, achieving something I couldn't dream of even three years ago. (See insert photos 6–11.)

WHAT ARE COMBINED TRANSPLANTS?

Dr. Walter Unger once said that only the most experienced and artistically best physicians could perform a transplant using all different types of transplant technology. Never has this been more true than in the late 90's. The experienced physician should be able to perform single-hair grafts for the hairline (you don't need a hairline in the middle of your head) as well as combine the best of all other processes in the same patient to achieve a superior result. He or she should be able to use slit grafts in female pattern hair loss, laser, and megasessions in those wanting thin but natural coverage, and linear in those desiring a natural yet thicker result.

Different patients have different needs. I had one gentleman who was totally bald but only wanted hair in the crown. When I asked him about the front, he simply said, "Bald fronts are sexy and I'm staying that way." Others have only asked for hair in the front of the bald scalp telling me that what they don't see doesn't bother them, and they don't see the backs of their heads.

So no matter how talented your doctor may be, he must listen to you. You won't wear his name on your head, just his result.

WHAT ABOUT THE DONOR AREA?

Over the years patients have brought in cartoons showing people post-transplant who now have a great resulting frontal head of hair. Then they turn around and you notice they now are bald in the back of the head. Well, years ago, we let the donor area close on its own, leaving small white scars where the hair was removed.

This pegboard effect could only be noticed if you lifted the hair in the donor area or if the hair was shaved closely. By the late 80's we started closing the donor area with sutures. This seemed to work because everyone has more skin than they need in the back of the head and suturing it closed seemed easy. The problems began with the big sessions where wide strips of hair were removed. In these cases, the closure was under tension, and the results were wide scars that we later had to revise.

Most doctors today know that too wide a strip of donor hair is a problem and thus would rather take a donor strip that's longer and thinner. By doing this, we are reducing the tension on the wound and allowing it to heal rapidly and with the thinnest of scar lines.

WILL THE DOCTOR REMOVE THE OLD SCARS FROM THE DONOR AREA?

Another valuable question to ask when interviewing a physician who may perform your procedure is, does he remove the old scars? By this I mean that a good physician will usually incorporate the scar of the previous donor area in the very corner of the next donor strip he removes. By doing this, when your transplant sessions are finished, you should wind up with only one thin scar in the donor area.

WILL TAKING DONOR MATERIAL CHANGE THE HEIGHT OF MY EARS OR SHORTEN MY NECK?

Patients often ask me during a consultation whether their ears move upward after enough donor is removed.

They don't!

I recently had another patient ask me if Ed Sullivan (the T.V. show host who introduced the Beatles to America) had a hair transplant. When I asked him why, he remarked that he thought so because the back of his neck seemed shorter than the front. I explained to him that we have so much extra skin in the back of our scalps that you'll never know it was removed.

The best way to visualize it is to think of people who shave their heads like Michael Jordan or Telly Savalas. You always see extra folds of skin in the back of the head. Your donor area consists of these folds. Also, cats carry their kittens by the back of the head because all mammals (including us) have extra skin there which is quite loose and easy to remove.

WHAT IF I HAD PREVIOUS TRANSPLANTS AND MY DONOR AREA WAS TAKEN THE OLD WAY?

Even if your donor area was plucked thoroughly and left with circles or no hair, we can now harvest (the medical term for remove) strips of donor. We simply use the good hair and discard the scars. We then cleanly sew the donor area back together and the result usually looks as good if not better than before you took the strip. The trick, once again, is long and narrow when removing the donor strips.

HOW QUICKLY WILL I HEAL?

Initial healing usually occurs in ten to twelve days. At first, most of the transplanted grafts will form small scabs. These are nature's protection for a healing area (just as you would get if you cut yourself shaving).

These scabs, as well as the sutures in the donor area, are ready to be removed in ten to twelve days. After removal, the healing of the graft sites is quick and very often indistinguishable after three weeks. In very bald scalps, camouflage (described elsewhere) can be applied, if necessary, after one or two days. In patients just thinning, combing their own hair over the transplant area works just fine.

The areas are healed and ready to receive additional transplants (if necessary) in six to eight weeks.

One of the most interesting changes resulting from the new transplant technology is the incredible healing in the recipient and donor sites. Because of this, even with magnification loops which I wear while performing transplants, I still can have difficulty seeing my prior work. It's not unusual for me to cancel a patient's second transplant procedure and wait for the hair to begin to grow before proceeding with another session. And when the hair grows, it's generally soft and quite natural. The plug look is just about gone.

IS THE PROCEDURE SAFE?

Part of interviewing your prospective doctor should include questions about instruments and sterility. Your doctor should have a hospital-type autoclave (sterilizer) and should have special disposal systems for medical waste.

The doctor and his technical staff should all have current Federal Occupational Safety Hazard Association (OSHA) certification and training.

A hair transplant is a clean procedure (hair can't be sterilized) but all instruments *must be!* Ask for a tour of your doctor's lab and ask to speak to one or several of his assistants. Do not be shy here! We all want hair, but we want it safely.

WHAT ARE THE DANGERS OF SURGERY?

A hair transplant is a minor surgical procedure, but it is still surgery. The main risks of this form of surgery fall into two categories—medical and aesthetic. Medical risks are about the same as that of dental procedures—namely bleeding and infection.

Medical Risks

Bleeding

When we first started performing transplants, we never sutured the donor area. As such, we would put pressure dressings as well as special clotting powders (like those used for cuts on boxers during fights) to seal the area. This worked fairly well, but we still had times when bleeding would occur after the procedure. We made ourselves available twenty-four hours a day for this, and fortunately it occurred in less than 2 percent of patients, but it can and did occur. Simple pressure would control the problem most of the time.

Now we use a form of laser technology to seal bleeding vessels in the donor area and then suture the area closed. This virtually eliminates the problem.

The recipient area rarely has any bleeding unless an accident occurs, and bleeding here is easily controllable with pressure.

Over the years, I have heard the craziest of accidents post-transplant.

Recently, I had a patient call me with bleeding on top of his head three days after his transplant. When I asked how it happened, he told me he was in a pet store with his friend and a loose monkey jumped on his head. Fortunately the damage was minimal.

Another patient had a garage door close on his head.

A father and son team played in a softball league one week after their transplants and got into a fight with the opposing team. They were both beaned with baseball bats.

Many patients have had their children pull their hair soon after transplants.

One patient went skiing, fell, and the ski came off and hit his head.

My favorite is three lawyers who came together for transplants and were driving home afterwards in their rented limousine. The limo was hit by a car and all three banged their heads together. When Emergency Medical Services arrived on the scene, they were confused as to who had already treated and bandaged the patients before they (EMS) arrived.

Other Causes of Bleeding

Rarely, patients would form a small blood blister (A-V malformation) during healing in the donor area. This would occur because the donor was left to heal on its own and occasionally two small blood vessels would heal together (an arteriole and a vein). This would form a small pulsating blood blister because the wall of the vein is thin and would expand like a small balloon when blood filled it.

I had one patient who was having a torrid love affair and his girlfriend stuck her fingernail right into his blood blister. He immediately started bleeding and she started screaming. His blood dripped on her and he thought he had injured her because he didn't feel any pain himself. The result was the police being called by concerned neighbors and an embarrassing trip to the hospital (he and she were at the height of lovemaking). He had two stitches and they went home red-faced.

The use of laser technology and suturing of donor has virtually eliminated this problem in most modern doctors' offices.

Infection

The scalp rarely gets infected. Old military manuals (circa 1950's and 60's) will advise medics that they don't even need gloves to sew up or treat scalp injuries. This is because the scalp has such a good blood supply that the body's defenses easily prevent infection from setting in. Today, doctors all wear gloves as protection for both the patient and physician.

Infection after a hair transplant is rare and is usually confined to a small area in the recipient site. It usually results from a zealous patient playing with his new grafts by picking off the scabs. This implants foreign dirt from under the fingernails causing a pimple and surrounding skin infection. It responds quickly and favorably to antibiotics and is rarely a problem. Infection after hair transplant occurs in less than 2 percent of patients in our practice. We always place patients on preventative antibiotics after treating them and have them return for followup in seven to ten days. We encourage them to call with questions and if in doubt, bring them into the office for a checkup.

Your doctor should not charge for checkups or stitch removals, although some do.

Aesthetic Risks

Placing aside bleeding and infection, a poor result can be the biggest risk in hair transplantation. The most common problems that I see are as follows.

Lack of Density

In their quest for a more natural result, many doctors have swung the pendulum too far and have decided to use only micrografting. This may be suitable for those who are looking for a thin, yet more natural result, but it can be devastating for those who expected a good amount of hair and wound up paying thousands for a "see-through" look. Ads have popped up showing dramatic results in seven months after one giant megasession of 2000+ grafts. When you examine the patient (as I have) you realize just how misleading photography can be. When you see these patients, you realize that there are no miracle results in short periods of time. I recently performed a transplant on a hairdresser who was disgusted after his third megasession. From a front view it didn't look bad until he tilted his head downwards. The patient started wearing a neck brace to prevent himself from accidentally bending over and allowing people to see how little hair he had. He looks better now and recently won a role in a major motion picture.

Fortunately, lack of density is usually treatable.

Hairline Too Low

This is a real problem. Several months ago I had a consultation with a young man and his father. The twenty-three-year-old prospective patient would not remove his hat until I locked the door to the consultation room to prevent anyone from accidentally entering. I've seen a lot in twenty-plus years, but his was the worst. When he took his hat off, he had a true Eddie Munster hairline. It was thick, black, and just above his eyebrows in a point. Normally I can adjust low hairlines by either removing some grafts or sending the patient for electrolysis, but this was hopeless. The patient had gone to a "weekend seminar" transplant expert and admitted that he had asked for a low hairline. But what if someone came to me and asked for me to cut their arm off? Sure I could do it, but it certainly is not good medicine. And neither was this. We wound up sending the patient out to California to be enrolled in an experimental new procedure to remove hair with little scarring. The results have yet to come in.

The caveat here is—keep the hairline higher, you can always easily lower it later on. We all will age and the maturity of the hairline must match the maturity of age.

Cornrow Hairline

This is usually the product of old transplant procedures or inexperience. It generally involves doctors forgetting that hairlines don't go from desert to forest. We all have a little buffer zone (even Ronald Reagan) and this is what makes the hairline look natural. Because of new technology, this is an easy correction. I can tell you it works because I now comb my hair straight back after years of covering my hairline. Single hairs and linear grafting have made the difference.

Cobblestoning

One of the big complications with the old plugs was the elevation of the individual grafts (actual bumps). This occurred because the grafts were always a bit larger than the receptor sites and thus they would not fit flush. Instead they would bulge like a cobblestone street. We were afraid in certain cases of trimming the grafts before inserting them because this could damage the hair follicles and thereby reduce hair growth. What we would do instead was trim the top of the graft, thereby flattening it. We always wait for several months, though, because often many of the grafts would flatten themselves over time.

In 1985, I published a paper where I demonstrated that by angling the grafts obliquely to the surface of the scalp, they would fit flush and the hair would grow in the proper direction.

Please remember, the longest distance between two points is on a diagonal rather than straight down. This simple adjustment helped prevent cobblestoning.

People with prior transplants with bumpiness can be helped now, as before, with a simple shaving of the surface of the graft. Because the roots are below the surface, they will not be harmed by this. This amounts to simple dermabrasion of the scalp. The hair will immediately begin to grow again after the correction is made.

Frizziness

Hair which has been transplanted may not always grow with the same texture as the area from which it has been taken. This was especially true during the "plug" era where larger circular plugs of hair and their roots were placed into sites which were narrower in diameter. This acted to squeeze the tissue tighter and caused the resulting hairs to grow frizzy. Much of this problem stopped when grafts stopped being condensed into smaller sites.

Subsequent studies have also shown that in some cases,

even with the most gentle care, the hair texture will change. The reason remains unclear, but with proper conditioning, this does not become a problem in grooming.

Doughnut Effect

This was definitely a function of the old round plugs. Some patients would develop a thin white circular area. Although this did not matter as much in areas of the scalp hidden by hair, it did matter when it occurred along the hairline.

Today's transplanted grafts rarely have this problem. In the case of prior ones which do, single-hair grafting or linear grafting through the white borders effectively eliminates the problem.

Misdirected Hair Grafts

Many of us remember Alfalfa in "Our Gang Comedies." This boy had a trademark cowlick that would not sit flat. Although some of us are born with misdirected hair in spots (cowlicks), others unfortunately have it created by the inexperienced transplant surgeon. Hair grows in specific directions on the front and vertex (crown) of the head. It is vital that transplanted hair grafts be directed to follow these directions.

In 1985 I published a method of "tunneling" of the recipient sites to help achieve this result. It's still in use today.

One of the odd situations I recall is a patient who came, not for a transplant, but for a cowlick repair. He had lived his thirty-two years with a patch of white hair that grew in the wrong direction in the front center of his hairline. He wanted it removed and replaced with hair with his normal color and direction of growth. The procedure worked perfectly.

Transplanted Grafts Spaced Too Far Apart

One of the biggest mistakes of the inexperienced transplant surgeon is placing the transplanted hair grafts far apart in an effort to cover more area. This is a real problem because once a fair number of grafts are placed in a bald area, the patient is committed to finishing the transplant in that area. Unlike zoysia grass, which are plugs of grass which grow together, transplanted grafts grow where they are positioned and only there. Now we run into the problem of filling in the in-between areas to make them look acceptable and this can be a devastating task.

So if you are fairly bald, concentrate on finishing the front half first. This way you are assured of a completed result in that area rather than a half complete job over the whole bald scalp.

Poor Growth

You can't transplant a tree by breaking off a branch and sticking it in the soil. Similarly, you can't transplant hair by moving the shafts and not the roots—they won't grow.

The most common cause of poor growth is technique. If a doctor removes the donor area properly, he should have taken the hairs out at the proper angles to preserve the roots. If he ignores the fact that hair grows at different angles from the scalp and that the roots are parallel to the shafts of hair, he can transect the roots causing little or no hair growth.

Having the grafts placed too close together can also cause poor growth. Blood supply initially feeds the grafts and promotes growth, but too many grafts in too small an area can decrease the hair yield per graft. This can also happen when a patient has transplant sessions very close together, not allowing enough time for healing and proper return of the blood supply.

A more recent problem occurs with megasessions. Here, subsequent sessions can cut the roots of previous transplanted hairs. In addition, the tediousness of properly dissecting thousands of individual hairs will often result in damage to hair.

Recently, articles have been published about the significant loss of roots of hairs after laser slits. A recent commentary by the editors of the *Journal of Cosmetic Surgery* reported up to a 50 percent hair loss.

To me, this is not acceptable.

Yes, not all grafts grow perfectly, but proper growth requires proper technique. Make sure your doctor has the experience to deliver.

Improper Donor Selection

When I begin a consultation, I always tell the prospective patient that a transplant is where we take hair from the sides and back of the head where it is never meant to fall out and transplant it to the bald or balding area on the top of the scalp. This is, of course, true in general. The specifics concern what is proper donor selection.

In someone over the age of forty with little recent additional hair loss, I am more liberal with donor selection than in someone who is twenty-one. Donor must be chosen with the future in mind. Hair transplantation is skin grafting. The skin (scalp in our case) always retains the characteristics of the area it comes from as long as it is placed on the same person or an identical twin (I have tried this successfully). It doesn't know it's been moved. If the donor selected has been taken too high, then when the twenty-one-year-old balds into that area in the future, he will also lose the hair taken from that area and transplanted to the balding scalp. Too often I see forty-year-old men come in with old exposed donor areas and thin results because someone chose an inappropriate area to take the hair from when the patient was young.

Other donor problems involve the location in which we wish to position the new hair. Hair that is closer to the lower sides of the head is generally thinner and should be used for hairlines. Hair from the center back of the head is good for central areas we wish to thicken. Neck hair is generally not good because it grows wispy and can be subject to later thinning with progressive hair loss.

HOW DO I CHOOSE A DOCTOR?

Choosing the right doctor for you requires some background leg work.

First, ask yourself, what you are looking to achieve as a result? What are your finances? Do you know others who have had transplants?

These are all questions which will help you in your interviews. Make sure you have them written down so you don't forget them in the nervousness of the consultation.

Choosing the right doctor should never be predicated on price. There are some that say "you get what you pay for." This is not true. The new doctors in the field, the clinics who advertise and market extensively, and the "elitists" may all charge more than they are worth.

I've had many patients come in to the office after spending ten to thirty thousand dollars for a poor result. First they tell me they went to the best, the ______ Medical Group. I ask them who performed their transplants, and most of the time they have no idea. I then ask them who advised and evaluated them during the consultation and they tell me it was a sales consultant. I often compare this to a dental secretary telling me I need caps and scheduling me for the procedure without ever consulting the dentist—it's dumb. It's okay to talk to a medical technician when the doctor is in surgery, but wait and speak to the physician as well. Make sure the doctor is not a "hired gun" for a layman-owned organization.

Referrals are a wonderful way to know what to do, but they are not always available to you. The next best thing is to ask to speak and even meet some of the doctor's patients. We all have patients who love to speak to others who once were in their situation. Don't be shy, take advantage of it.

Another smart idea is to sit in the waiting room for a bit and talk to ongoing patients—here you will generally learn the facts.

Pictures are wonderful, but make sure they are compatible—in other words, don't compare a before shot taken with a Polaroid flash to an after shot taken with no flash in a dark setting. Also, ask to see top views of the head before and after, not just side and frontal views which may hide the whole picture. We saw a clear example of this in the before and after megasession photos on page 3 of the insert.

Ask what other procedures the doctor performs and learn how many transplants he or she performs weekly. I had one patient who went to the chairman of surgery of a major teaching center to have his hernia repaired. He thought this guy must be the best! When the operation failed, he learned that the chairman had rarely performed hernia surgery in the past few years. He would have done better with the community surgeon—but he went for stature over experience. Look for both.

Calling various organizations can help as well. But be careful, some charge doctors to be listed and the requirement to be recommended is paying the price. Look at the American Hair Loss Council, the American Academy of Cosmetic Surgery, the American Society for Dermatologic Surgery, and your local medical societies to check on the credentials of the doctor. Call the local Better Business Bureau to judge complaints. All of us have someone we didn't agree with, but few of us have a large number.

Finally, if you are unsure, ask for a test session. This involves transplanting a few grafts from the donor to a carefully chosen recipient site, usually in the back or side of the head near the remaining hair. Photograph the sites where they are placed and then watch for yourself both healing and growth—if you like it then go ahead with that doctor.

It took you a long time to lose the hair, you can wait a few months to make sure the replacement is what you want. I have numerous patients who give me every excuse why they have to delay a second session—but I know they want to see the result before they proceed. When I bring it up to them on the reevaluation, they usually deny it at first, but eventually they all "come clean."

It's okay to see if you're happy before you proceed; it's your head!

WHAT ARE SOME OF THE FALSE PROMISES PEOPLE MIGHT HEAR?

Although I touched on this earlier, it's best to answer this question here. I talk with twenty to thirty prospective patients each week. Many of them have been elsewhere before sitting down with me. First, they are usually surprised to see me because at many of the other hair transplant facilities they've gone to, they only talked with a sales consultant and not the doctor.

Of all the false promises that I hear made elsewhere (usually not by the doctor but by the sales associate), the most common is that in one large session you can have a thick full head of hair. It just doesn't happen that way. It sounds great because you may wish it's true, but honestly, no doctor can achieve density of growth plus naturalness in one giant session. Hair transplantation is an art, art requires refinement, and refinement takes time.

Another false promise is that you can go out for dinner the night after surgery or return to work right after your procedure. This may be minor surgery, but it is surgery and surgery requires physical rest for one or two days at least. You may feel well at the end of the procedure, but resting afterwards is the smartest and safest way to go. If you must go out, avoid physical exertion.

My favorite false promise is you'll have your hair back in six months. The hair (as I discussed before) generally takes three months to start growing. The second session generally takes place two to four months later. So at six months, the first session will have about 1½ inches of growth and the second will just be sprouting.

I always tell patients, "You won't get a head of hair overnight, but when you do, it will last a lifetime." Be patient! I remember one distraught couple that came to see me about her fiancé's hair. He had a hat on. They had gone to a clinic based in Canada who promised him that he would look good for his wedding in five months. The patient had told them that, if not, he would rather have his transplant after the wedding. Well, after believing what he was told by the hair consultant, he had a transplant in just mildly thinning frontal hair (I saw his before pictures). The result was hair shock (see prior section) and rapid thinning of his surrounding hair. The wedding was in one month and they were thinking of cancelling it. Calls to his doctor in Canada went unanswered.

What I did was have a partial clip-in hairpiece made for him (cost, three hundred dollars). Here he was able to add just enough hair unnoticeably that he was able to walk about without his hat. He got married, went to Aruba on his honeymoon, and months later proceeded slowly with me to fill in other thinning areas.

One last false promise is "Do it now and you'll never need to do it again." This is only true if you have finished your balding process. I don't perform preventative transplants. I can't tell you how many young men want me to just shave their heads and fill every spot in, hair there or not. Some come in with their heads already shaven. No responsible physician will transplant into a good hair growth area to get it over with. If you lose more hair in the future, you may need more transplants. I just had an additional transplant session after sixteen years (I had thinned more in the back). The beauty was that my prior transplanted hair easily covered the newest work and I suffered no personal detection even by close friends.

Although I'm sure there are many other minor ones, the above should help guide you into realizing that if something sounds too good, don't simply believe it.

DOES THE TRANSPLANT HAIR ALWAYS TAKE AND FOR HOW LONG WILL IT LAST?

This question is as common as "Does it hurt?" The answer is, if done properly by an experienced physician, it will generally always take (maybe not always at 100 percent as I have described previously) and will grow for the rest of your life plus two weeks (hair and nails grow for two weeks after we depart).

Remember, the hair lasts as long on the same person in the new area as it did where it came from. So if the donor area was selected properly, it will continue to grow in the previously bald sites.

Occasionally, I will do test sessions on patients with previous scarring from injuries, burns, prior radiation therapy hair loss, or hair loss secondary to disease or surgery. Although it usually works, I never risk the chance that it will not. This is one of the main values of test sessions.

IS THE TRANSPLANT NOTICEABLE?

I had a patient about eighteen years ago who was completely bald in the front (type IV). He was a pharmacist and was in the public eye. He realized that he wasn't going to be able to cover the fresh transplants (transplants were very obvious years ago) and so he decided that he rather just face the situation. He placed a piece of tape on his forehead with two arrows on it facing upwards with the words "hair transplant" between them. No one had the nerve to even question him about them.

Today, we have other methods of dealing with noticeability. We may use temporary hairpieces, or simply use the patients' remaining hair to camouflage the problem. Makeups and special creams are out there (see prior chapter), but I still have my loyal core of diehards who just don't care if people notice. One construction worker told me that if people ask what he's having done at least he knows he's transplanting his own growing hair, not gluing on a hair system. "It's not like they can ask me to take off my wig down the road. This is my own hair and if they don't like it—tough."

Many of us have become our own hairstylists. By this I mean we have learned creative combing to cover thinning or bald areas. Hair spray has become the tool of choice in helping combat the common enemy—the gust of wind.

About ten years ago Jack Anderson, a columnist for the *New York Times*, wrote an editorial about the value of hair spray in covering the bald spots of our elected officials in Congress. His comment was that congressmen and senators have to be careful when climbing the capital building steps so they won't fall down and break their hairdos.

The same creativity that is used to cover bald spots can easily be helpful in covering the fresh transplants (along with cosmetics if necessary). The small clip-in hair addition has proven to be inexpensive, simple to apply, and great as a temporary cover for those who need something extra to fill the spot. I used one in 1975, and by keeping it high and then combing natural hair over it, nobody could tell I was wearing it unless they ran their fingers through my hair(piece).

The key changes in recent years is the rapid and almost complete healing of the grafts. The modern small or narrow linear or laser grafts heal quickly with minimal scabbing and rapid return of natural skin color. Patients no longer have circular red spots for twelve weeks, making the need for camouflage now very temporary.

Sun and salt water has proven an aid for rapid healing. Unlike other forms of cosmetic surgery where you're instructed to stay out of the sun for six months, sun and salt water speed the healing of hair transplants rapidly. Because of this, many of my patients will have a transplant right before going to a warm sunny climate to rest and heal. After my last procedure, which I had on a Thursday evening I went to Mexico on Sunday. I arrived at the hotel at 5 p.m. and immediately changed and dove into the ocean. One week later, when I returned home, the scabs were gone and the grafts blended in perfectly with my surrounding scalp.

I have other patients who in the winter months will go to the beach just to fill their spray bottles with salt water. They are convinced (and so am I) that natural brine works the best.

AM I TOO OLD FOR A TRANSPLANT?

When asked this question, I often tell people the story of my oldest patient. He was eighty-two, a recent widower, and wanted hair so he would look younger and date women in their 60's. The transplant worked well (gray hair blends great with the scalp) and at ninety-six this patient is still going strong (yes, the hair is still there). I only transplanted the front of his scalp but he looks great with the hair combed back.

My youngest patient was an eleven year-old girl who had a big scar on the crown of her head from a traumatic forceps delivery. I actually performed scalp reductions on her and only used a few grafts along the reduction suture line to finish it. She still sends me holiday cards with a picture each year.

What I'm trying to say is that if someone is healthy, age is not a problem when performing hair transplants. Yes, I modify the approach in the older patient, but there is no such thing as "over the hill" in this field.

Last year I performed additional work on an eighty-year-old man who had his transplants begun in California. The man had a huge red birthmark on his forehead. When I asked him what about seeing someone to treat the birthmark, his answer was "What birthmark?" In other words, when he looked in the mirror all he saw was hair loss and a good doctor treats what bothers the patient, not what bothers the physician.

The field of geriatric hair transplants has become so popular that it is now part of modern textbooks and the subject of many publications.

It especially has spiraled in Florida. Healing is as quick and complete in the elderly patient and the results are just as excellent. Of course, I always get medical clearance first from the patient's physician and insist on both the patient seeing him and my speaking with him before any procedure.

WHO IS A CANDIDATE FOR TRANSPLANTS?

When I talk with a prospective patient I often investigate the following.

1. What are his concerns about his hair loss?
2. What are his expectations?

This is important because a person with good donor area and a reasonable amount of hair loss may be a bad candidate if he expects unrealistic results. I remember one young patient who came into the office with this giant thick hairpiece on his head. First he bet me I was wondering why someone with so much hair would come to consult with me. I didn't want to tell him how obvious and absurd the hairpiece looked, and so I played along. When he removed the hairpiece (it was taped on) I acted shocked and told him that I now understood why he was here. I then asked him what type of result he was seeking. He told me he wanted nothing short of his childhood hairline and density. I encouraged him to keep the wig. In other words, he was a bad candidate for reasons other than strictly donor hair quality.

A good candidate is someone who is realistic about his goals based on his existing pattern of hair loss and remaining hair density. He or she understands that it will take time for the hair to grow and is willing to undergo several sessions if necessary to achieve the desired result. Hair transplantation is an art as well as a science, and art takes time and work. If the patient is young, a good candidate will allow the hairline to be a bit higher (in case of extensive baldness occurring in later years) and will understand that future sessions may be needed if further hair loss occurs.

The doctor and the patient are a team. Both should be patient and available to work together to achieve the desired result. Knowing this makes for a good candidate.

ARE HAIR TRANSPLANTS DIFFERENT FOR WOMEN THAN MEN?

As I've mentioned in an earlier chapter, there are two main types of genetic hair loss, male and female pattern

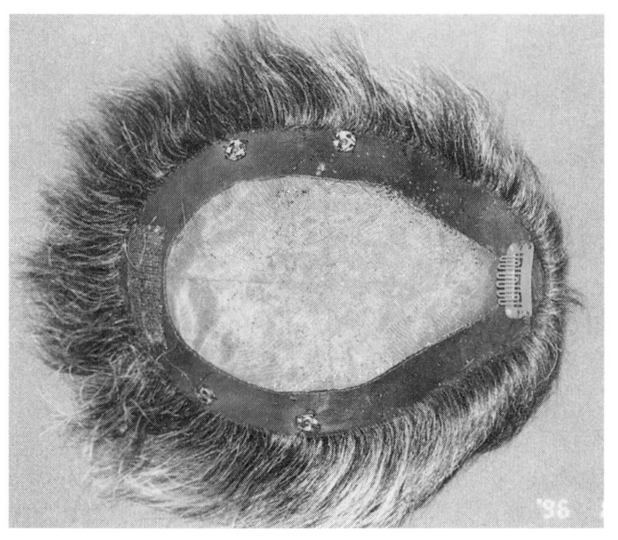

1

Hairpiece with clip

Gary S. *Hitzig*, M.D.

Great Cover-up
Applied to Thinning Hair

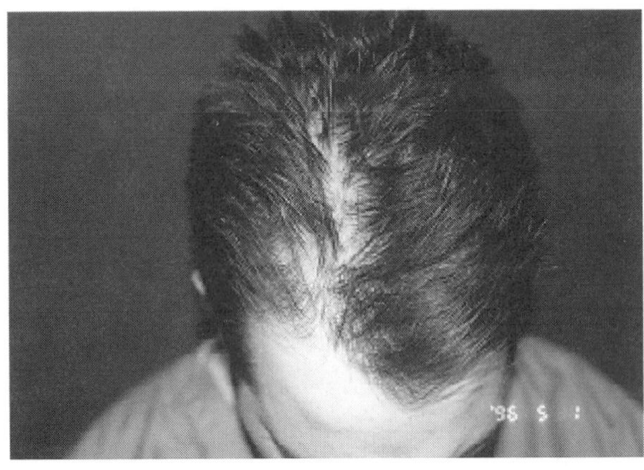

2

Before

More Hair Cosmetics, Inc.

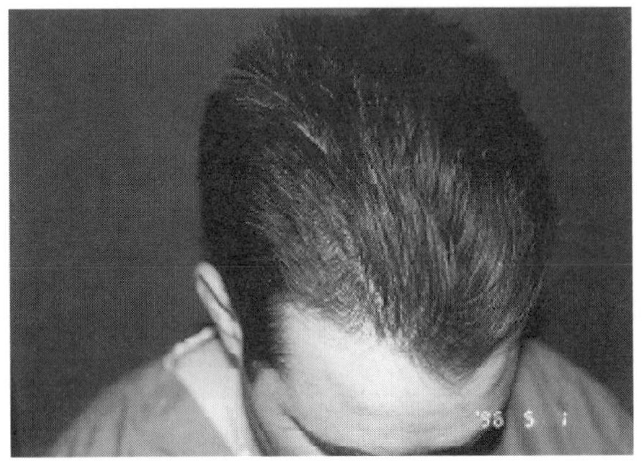

3

After

More Hair Cosmetics, Inc.

Megasession Results

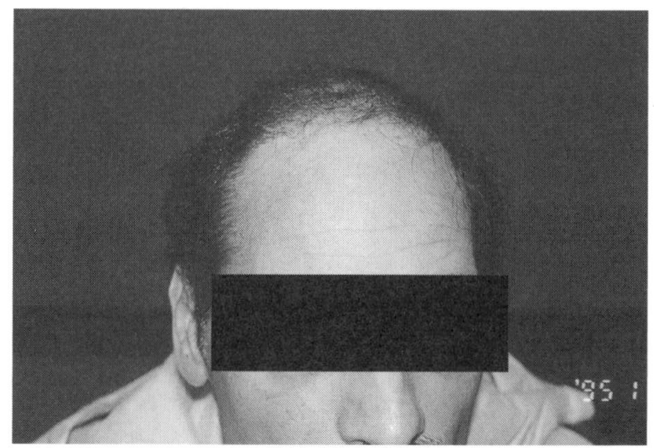

4

Front view

Gary S. *Hitzig*, M.D.

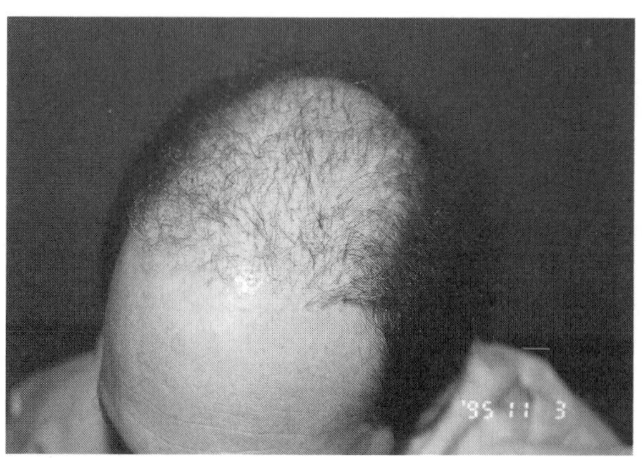

5

Top view. Note true thinness.

Gary S. *Hitzig*, M.D.

Linear Graft Transplant Sequence for a Caucasian Male

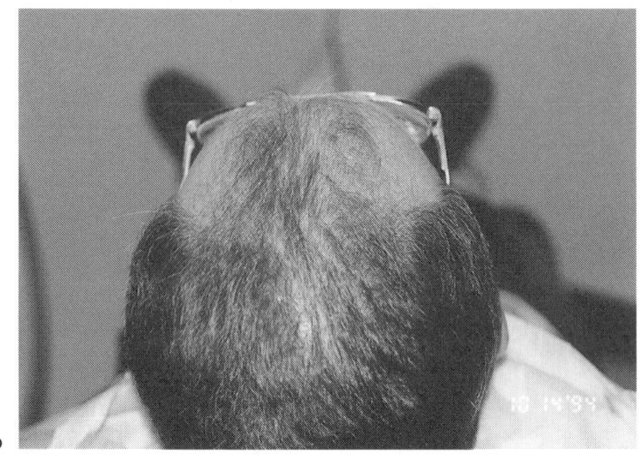

6

54-year-old patient prior to first session (top view)

Gary S. *Hitzig*, M.D.

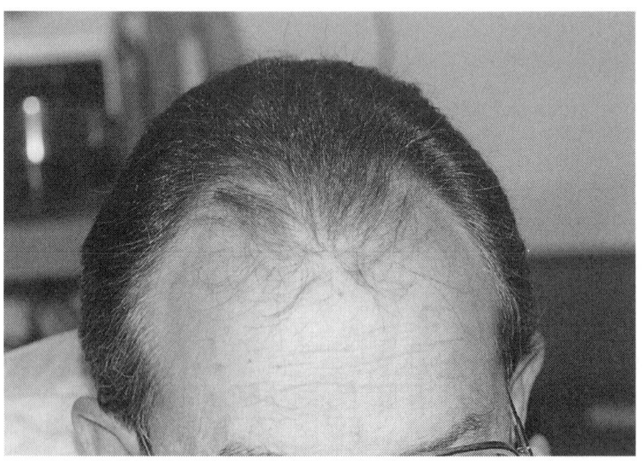

7

54-year-old patient prior to first session (front view)

Gary S. *Hitzig*, M.D.

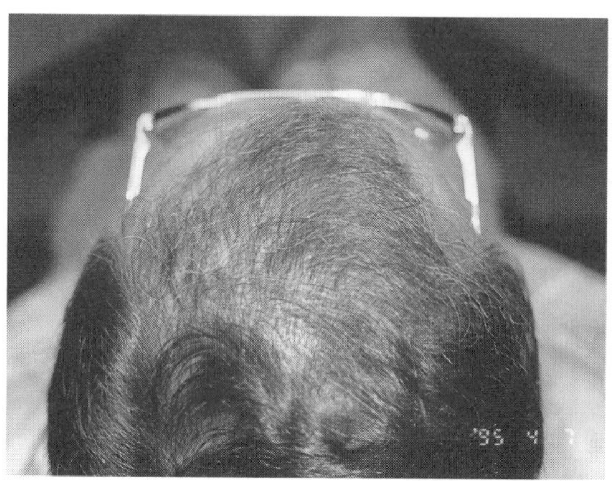

8

Same patient six months after first session (top view)

Gary S. Hitzig, M.D.

9

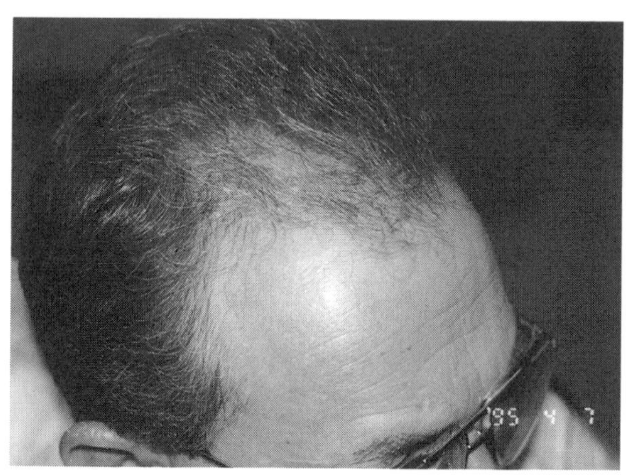

Same patient six months after first session (front view)

Gary S. Hitzig, M.D.

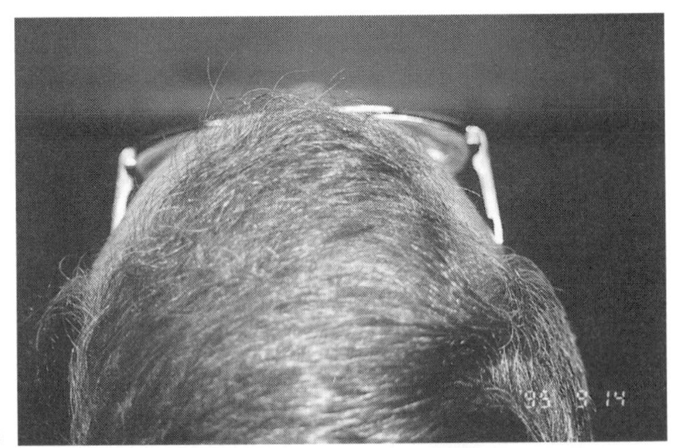

10

Same patient after two sessions with a total of 350 varying size linear grafts, eleven months after first session (top view)

Gary S. Hitzig, M.D.

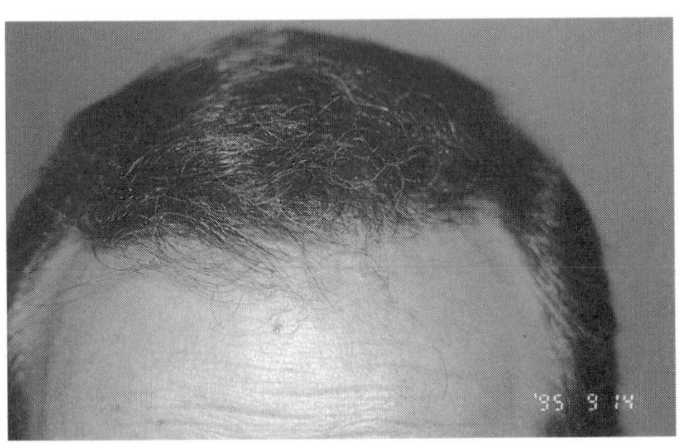

11

Same patient after two sessions with a total of 350 varying size linear grafts, eleven months after first session (front view)

Gary S. Hitzig, M.D.

Transplant in an African-American Male

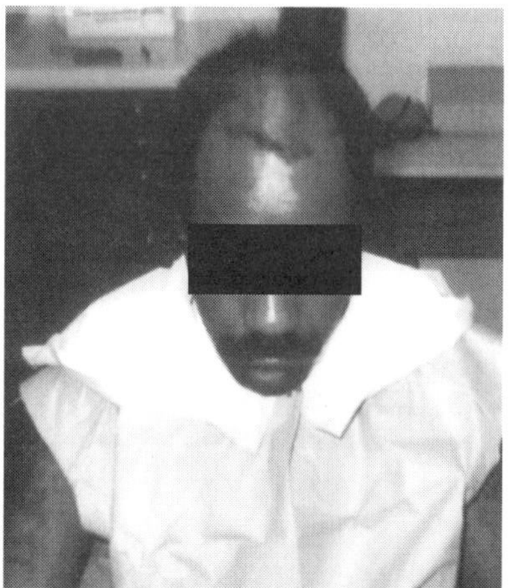

12

Before

Gary S. Hitzig, M.D.

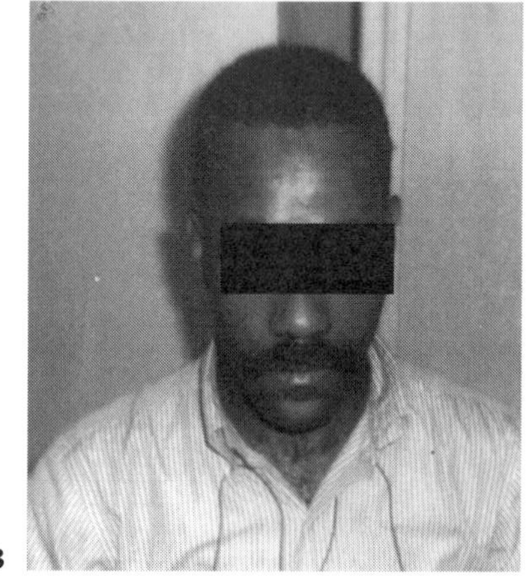

13

After

Gary S. Hitzig, M.D.

Schematic Drawing of Scalp Flap Technique

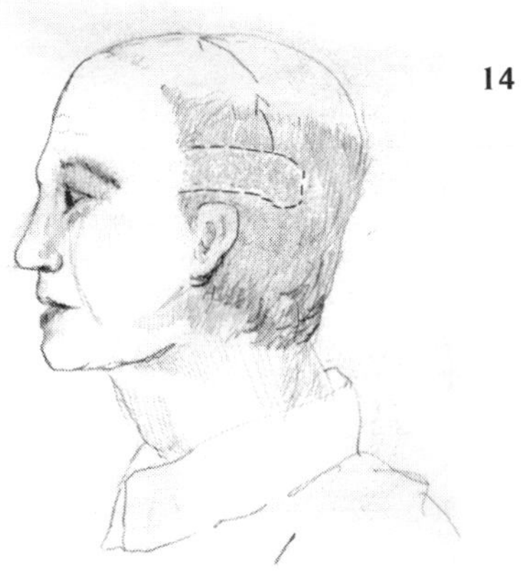

14

Before *Sue Lerner*

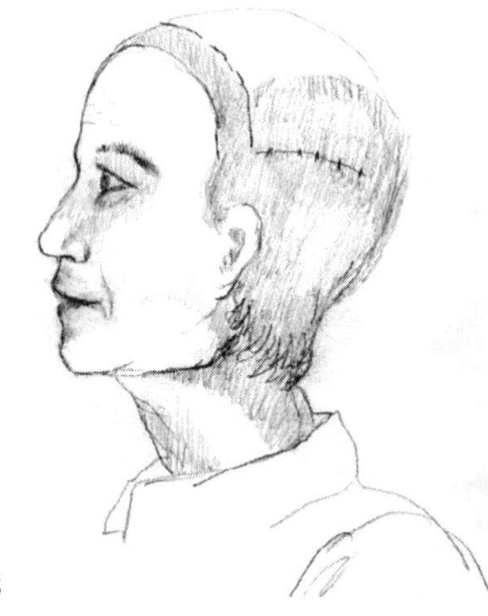

15

After. Note that hair grows in the wrong direction when the flap is in its final placement on top of the scalp.

Sue Lerner

alopecia. In male pattern baldness, we will often see a thinning area of the scalp progressing to near complete or complete hair loss in the affected area. In female pattern baldness, however, the loss is generally more subtle and the result is a generalized thinning of the hair in the affected area without ever becoming slick bald. This is called the *veil effect*.

Because of these distinctions, we wish in the male situation to replace the area of hair loss by removing and replacing bald with hair-bearing skin. In the classic female case, however, any removal of skin will be accompanied by the removal of some growing hair as well. Because of this, we choose to modify the type of transplant we will perform in female pattern hair loss.

Slit grafts and single hair insertions seem to work the best to thicken a thinning area. Over a year ago, I performed a transplant on a young Chinese pop artist who had originally had classic plugs to the front of her scalp performed in Taiwan. The transplant removed much of her own existing hair and as such, there was little improvement but substantial visibility now of the transplanted hair. I actually removed parts of the large plugs allowing them to ''decompress'' (spread out the hair to look softer), and then performed several hundred single-hair insertions to disguise the previous work and thicken the area. She now wears her hair tied back and looks great in her publicity photos.

For other women, by inserting slit grafts (no skin removed) you are essentially pushing the surrounding hair closer together and inserting thicker hair at intervals within the thinning area. The pitting and tufting of slits can be avoided as long as the grafts are not placed too close to each other and by placing the grafts slightly above the surface of the scalp. In the course of a few days, they then settle to scalp level and become flat. Growth commences anywhere from four to twelve weeks depending on how small the grafts are (single hairs grow quicker).

The most important point here is not to get too aggressive in the procedure and not to do repeat procedures sooner than four to six months. This is because repeat or aggressive procedures can "shock" the surrounding hair causing further loss. The use of minoxidil with the transplant and in the immediate weeks thereafter can substantially diminish the chance of hair shock. Injections of Kenalog (a local form of cortisone used in alopecia areata) can also be used to prevent and reverse hair shock.

If the above principles are followed, hair transplantation is indeed a valuable and viable option for women with female as well as many other types of hair loss.

ARE THERE DIFFERENT APPROACHES IN HAIR TRANSPLANTING FOR CAUCASIANS, AFRICAN-AMERICANS, AND ASIANS?

Although hair replacement surgery is most common today amongst Caucasions, it has been receiving increasing press and thus popularity amongst other major ethnic groups as well—notably African-Americans and Asians. Over ten years ago I was asked to appear on several news programs geared toward African-Americans. I was also interviewed by magazines such as *Ebony and Essence* in order to explain hair replacement surgery to black men (and women). The point was to create reader awareness of the procedure but to also warn African-Americans to avoid pitfalls specific to them.

More recently I have been interviewed by several Chinese newspapers who are focusing their efforts on informing their readers about hair replacement surgery. This is because traditionally hair loss amongst Asians is treated by hat, hairpiece, or synthetic hair, not hair transplantation. It is only now becoming more popular with many physicians in the Orient beginning to open medical practices devoted solely to hair replacement. Here, too, the special needs to modify procedure to adjust for coarse straight dark hair on lighter skin requires an experienced touch to perform a successful procedure.

WHAT ARE THE CONCERNS SPECIFIC TO AFRICAN-AMERICANS?

Keloid scarring is an abnormal healing of cuts whereby wide, distorted, and elevated scarring results rather than a thin healing line. Even minor cuts in those who have a propensity to keloid can become obvious and unsightly. I have seen women who pierce their ears wind up with large "balls" of scar tissue at the puncture site. Keloiding is thought to be genetically transmitted.

Keloid scarring occurs in about 5–7 percent of African Americans. Yet when it occurs, it can be devastating to the patient and until recently, almost impossible to treat. Therefore, the fear of keloiding has been instrumental in slowing the enthusiasm for hair replacement surgery in this ethnic group.

We have learned over the course of time, however, that even those blacks who keloid on other parts of the body rarely scar on the scalp. This is because the scalp has such wonderful blood supply allowing quick healing with little complication. In all blacks with a history of keloid scarring, I routinely perform a small test session usually in the rear in an area that's not obvious near adjacent good hair growth to prove to both the patient and myself that keloiding will not be a problem.

As such keloiding has not been a problem, however there are other differences your doctor must be aware of and deal with if you are African-American and your procedure is to have the best chance of success.

Hair in blacks grows at different angles than whites. The hair shaft usually arises perpendicular to the scalp surface. This is important if your doctor is to avoid cutting off the roots when creating his donor strip. In addition, the grafts themselves are more technical to prepare as the hairs from the root to scalp surface bow (curve) rather than grow straight as in other groups. This can lead to cutting of many of the hair roots unless the preparer is experienced in dealing with African-American hair.

Another problem is follicle depth. Often the hair roots in the donor area are very deep while the recipient area is shallower. The inexperienced or unprepared transplanter can cause cobblestoning (see the complications of hair transplants) if he doesn't prepare his recipient sites at the right angle to compensate for this.

Depigmentation of the skin (whitish color of grafts after transplantation) was a problem back when doctors used big plugs. The smaller grafts do not seem to cause this problem. Occasionally tattooing was needed to deal with this successfully in the past.

Hair density in African-Americans is far less than in Caucasians. As a result the grafts need to be placed closer together to insure the hair to be able to coil and mesh with the surrounding hairs.

Finally, donor hair strips must be thinner in blacks than whites. This is because wider strips tend to scar more readily in blacks. It is better here to take longer thinner strips to maximize your result without challenging healing.

When the above parameters are followed, your results can be quite dramatic and cosmetically superior. (See insert photos 12–13.)

WHAT ARE THE CONCERNS SPECIFIC TO ASIANS?

In the past few years the numbers of people of Asian descent that I have transplanted have increased dramatically. Here, as with blacks, hair type and density come into play.

It seems that Asians have less hair density than whites but more than blacks. The more important consideration is that Asian hair is generally straight and black. Asian skin is often pale compared to their hair color. This combination of straight dark hair on pale skin makes bad hair replacements stick out like a sore thumb. In Asians, the old plugs just didn't work. The newer techniques, however, work well. A larger zone of single hairs in the frontal hairline, part, and crown are needed as well as considerable densifications with additional grafts placed between any areas previously transplanted into. Linear grafting has worked very well by helping to eliminate gaps between prior hair transplant grafts, even the old plugs, while still providing good density of growth. Prior patients have even resorted to tattooing or synthetic hair implants between transplanted hair to encourage the appearance of hair density and avoid the unsightly contrast of dark hair and pale skin.

No responsible physician should just go ahead and transplant any patient who asks for it, but this is especially true for African-Americans and Asians. If you are either, you owe it to yourself to see and talk to other patients in your ancestral category, no matter what it may be. Don't believe that a lot of experience with other forms of surgery or hair transplantations in Caucasians alone qualifies your doctor to transplant you if you are not. You have to be your own best advocate. Check their experience. Then check their results.

ARE MY ACTIVITIES RESTRICTED BEFORE MY TRANSPLANT?

Prior to having a transplant, there are several general precautions that most doctors will take. Further specifics are usually given prior to the transplant procedure. Typical preoperative instructions include the following.

- Do not get a haircut prior to a transplant because any trimming required will be done by the hair transplant technician. If the hair is cut too close, the doctor may not be able to determine where to put the transplants. Also, shampoo your hair well as close to the hair transplant time as possible. Even though we will place an antiseptic on the ear, it's nicer to start with a clean scalp.
- Eat a good meal during the day, but do not eat or drink anything within one hour prior to scheduled transplant. This is because hungry people are more nervous. The one-hour period not to eat is to prevent nausea during nitrous oxide anesthesia.
- Do not exercise twenty-four hours prior to transplant. Exercise tends to raise blood pressure temporarily. This usually increases the chance of bleeding during the procedure.

- Wear a shirt which buttons rather than a pullover as your head may have a small dressing. If you have a hairpiece, you will not be able to wear it until the second day.
- It is important that no alcoholic consumption takes place within forty-eight hours of transplant surgery. Alcohol interferes with your blood platelets and slows down the clotting process.
- Do not take any aspirin or aspirin-containing products for the same reason you shouldn't drink alcohol.
- Don't forget to write down your questions for the doctor before the procedure. This is because nervousness may make you forget to have your concerns answered at the time. Write the answers down so you will remember them.

ARE MY ACTIVITIES RESTRICTED AFTER MY TRANSPLANT?

The biggest restrictions after a transplant involve no heavy physical activity for five to seven days. This is usually the most contested instruction, as most people feel fine after the procedure. Nevertheless, the first place that gets robbed of circulation when you're active is the skin and scalp. Blood gets diverted to the muscles; blood pressure rises, and people bang their transplanted area. Any surgery, even minor, requires rest afterwords, this is no different.

Don't drink alcohol or take aspirin for forty-eight hours for the same reason as before.

Postoperative medicines are prescribed, and in some cases, such as with tetracycline and/or minoxidil with Retin

A, they can restrict your ability to go out in direct sunlight.

Swelling is a normal and harmless occurrence following the transplant and usually occurs two to four days from the date of surgery. In order to avoid swelling around the eyes when doing the transplant in the frontal area, lie back as much as possible and apply a cool compress to your forehead every two to three hours for fifteen minutes. If swelling comes down into the forehead, work the swelling to the side with your fingers, and apply a warm compress to your forehead. If prescribed, taking Motrin 400mg tabs four times daily will help prevent swelling as well. The doctor in some cases will have injected you with Kenalog (a type of cortisone) to help prevent swelling. Prednisone tablets with decreasing dosage over a six-day period may be provided as well for the same reason.

The grafts and the donor area should be cleansed thoroughly with alcohol first upon removal of the dressing, and three times daily thereafter for two weeks. Do not apply alcohol to the crusts for five days if you have "flexible collodian." (No bandage but a clear protective sealant instead.)

Remember to drench the gauze sponge with alcohol and to pat or dab on the alcohol—do not rub.

Do not pick at the scabs—let them fall off. Extreme care must be exerted so that your comb or brush does not catch on the scabs during the healing process.

You may shampoo your hair on the third day. While shampooing, use only your fingertips. Apply alcohol at once to both grafts and donor area. Vitamin E oil can be applied at night to help promote healing after two weeks.

You can generally return to work in two or three days (this is why I'm so busy at the end of the week), but if the work requires heavy lifting, accommodations should be made.

In my experience, at the end of seven to ten days, there

are no further restrictions. The patients can resume all their prior activities in full. Now begins the waiting game, but rest assured, if your procedure was performed by a competent surgeon and you've followed his instructions, your hair will grow.

HOW MUCH WILL IT COST?

There was an old statement that "if you have to ask the price, you can't afford it." This may have been true for diamonds and jewelry which are nice luxuries, but not the biggest necessity, but it is not true for hair replacement surgery.

In the past, we used to charge per plug. This was because we generally used a standard size plug and transplanted thirty to one hundred plugs per session. The average price was fifteen to one hundred dollars per plug depending on the doctor. Today, price per transplant graft can be deceiving. A graft can have ten hairs, or it can have one hair. Sessions of several hundred to several thousand grafts are common.

Because of this, most responsible doctors now charge per session. You come to us with a bald area to fill, it's our responsibility to try to accomplish this to the best of our ability. Often I will have patients who are on a budget. If I charge per graft and find I need more grafts per session, the price would become prohibitive.

Remember, when you compare prices or see a low price per graft advertised, you may be comparing apples to oranges. Three thousand single-hair grafts at three to six dollars each is no bargain—that's between nine and eighteen thousand dollars per session. Compare results and numbers of hairs transplanted—it makes things clearer.

In my office, a typical session will range from fifteen hundred to four thousand dollars depending on the amount of bald area to be covered. I typically perform two large sessions on a patient and then wait six months to reevaluate both the results and the need for further work. I often wait this period because the grafts heal so well I have trouble locating them even with magnifying loops. Also, by allowing the hair to grow first, any remaining area that needs to be transplanted will become obvious. Third sessions are generally half the price of the previous two. So in my hands, transplant costs range from three to ten thousand dollars in most cases. When asked why am I so reasonable, my answer is "I have been performing transplants for more than twenty years. Don't ask me why I'm so cheap; ask them why they're so expensive." Perhaps they don't perform too many of them.

Prices do cover a considerable range, though. People still charge up to twenty thousand dollars per session. This is especially true in the case of megasessions where they have a sliding scale of price per graft depending on the numbers.

Sometimes I think some doctors forget most of our patients are hardworking, decent people. I don't believe there is any reason to charge outrageous prices just, as one physician put it, "because I can get it." I grew up in a family where my father was a police officer and my mother stayed home to care for several of us. Although his priority was putting food on the table, he would go for a little luxury if the price was in his budget. Hair replacement surgery should be within your budget.

One doctor sends out information that you only get what you pay for. Don't believe it. You don't have to pay for fancy advertising, offices, and commissioned sales consultants, you should only pay for results.

CAN MY PREVIOUS TRANSPLANT BE REPAIRED?

About 35 to 40 percent of my patients have had previous transplants elsewhere. This is up from 15 to 20 percent two years ago and probably results from all the novices and hot shots who have entered the field. In general, your transplant can be refined with today's technology. I, myself, had a whole new hairline transplanted, and I also densified my prior transplant with both single and linear grafts. Retransplanting has been performed where the old thick hairline plugs are divided in half, leaving one half in place and moving the other half to another area in order to soften the effect. Prior donor areas that we thought were "picked clean" have been reutilized and old scars have been revised.

I had one patient who was a computer whiz (he started a big portion of the Internet). He had had prior transplants ten years ago and had lost some more hair. In his conversation, he asked me, in computer terms, whether we could upgrade his p.a. (personal appearance). My answer to him and to you is that transplants are upgradeable. You don't have to wait twenty years for the ultimate procedure, your doctor only has to make sure he's left enough donor area to allow it to be performed in the future.

WHAT KIND OF RESULTS MIGHT I EXPECT?

The results you can expect are dependent on what you wish to achieve. For example, if you are just beginning to thin in the temple regions and wish to fill them in, this is indeed possible. The key is knowing that every bald space on the top of the head cannot be restored to its second-grade glory. Reality and expections must always be close.

The results you can achieve vary with the following.

Available Donor Area

If your donor area is thin (number of hairs per unit area), fine (texture of the hair), and straight, you are better off trying to achieve a thinner yet natural result. Lots of single hairs for the hairline zone are backed up with larger grafts (linear in my case) to give some additional density but still avoid any obvious transplant result. Work in the frontal area first and get this right before moving on to any bald area in the crown. You can always continue to thicken the front then and are not committing yourself to finishing another area. Lots of naturally balding men have thin zones in the crown area. Once you're satisfied with the frontal result, then sit with your doctor and discuss what can be achieved towards the crown.

If you are one of those 3 to 5 percent of people who bald excessively and have the Superdome on top, then you definitely want to stick with small grafts which, although thin, will still give the illusion of hair. First try some test transplants along your own hair border and make sure you're happy with the healing and growth. You may opt for a frontal forelock which diffuses the bald look in front and is yet natural or you may want to go slowly and see what you can ultimately achieve. I have three patients who were very bald as the representative pictures show in the photo insert, and who, over the course of two to three years (in conjunction with scalp reductions), have gone farther than I ever could have predicted. The key was we worked slowly and could have stopped at any time. The smaller grafts with single hairs in front plus some larger linear backup always kept it from looking like a transplant.

Donor Plus Age

When donor area is plentiful, thick, lighter-colored, and wavy, the sky is generally the limit. This is modified, however, by the age of the patient. If he is young, the experienced doctor is aware that he may bald excessively and will keep the hairline high, transplant only in the frontal region, and warn the patient of the need to be followed in the future. A good doctor will tell him clearly that he will *most probably* require additional transplants as the years go on. He will also not be swayed by the insistence of the patient to have a low hairline.

I had one young man who told me he would sign a consent form for me to transplant a low hairline. My answer was "I know better, and even if you give me permission, it is still wrong and I won't do it." It's better to lose a patient here than to live with the consequences of the mistake, even if the patient wants to take responsibility for it.

Hair Color

Light hair on a light skin background hides a multitude of sins. This was the basis for the "spray on hair in a can" we all saw on late night T.V.

What the eye tends to notice is contrast. So if you have dark hair and light skin, the bald spots become obvious. I often tell blond-haired men and women that if they dyed their hair black, they would immediately look balder.

Well this is an advantage in the patient with light skin

and blond or light brown hair, or dark skin with dark brown or black hair.

When the skin and hair color come close, your result can be superior. Even thinner grafts will appear to grow thicker to the eye, and the hairline becomes an easy job to make virtually natural.

If the donor is plentiful, you can expect to cover even a type V or VI baldness to a very natural satisfactory degree. You can proceed quicker with your transplant with little worry of it being detectable, even in the early stages.

If the hair is dark and curly and the skin pale, proceed slower but rest assured, most of you can achieve the appearance of full coverage on the top. Once again this is restricted by your age, available donor, your patience, and your treating physician. Always ask to see results and talk to other patients first. And remember, each of us is different—you must talk with *your physician* (not a hair consultant) and review what the possibilities are for you.

Expectations and Results

It all comes back to this. You must work with your hair. Your natural hair (before you lost it) required care and grooming, and so will your transplant. The doctor can only make it grow, you must take care of it.

I have had so many patients return after their hair grew in only to see them still parting their hair just above the ear. The hair looks silly this way. When I change the part, I show them how much better it looks. They don't need to comb their hair like they're bald anymore—they are not! Now I include a referral to a trained hairstylist with each transplant if the patient desires it. It's amazing what a little professional grooming can accomplish.

CAN I COMBINE HAIR TRANSPLANTS WITH HAIR SYSTEMS?

A recent CNN broadcast reported the increasing use of hair weaves and hairpieces in the movies (e.g. Sharon Stone in *Casino*). Although the actors and actresses have both hairstylists and makeup artists on the set to make sure these look like real growing hair, the average person does not have that luxury.

Several surveys, including a large one taken in my own practice, asked both men and women what they felt made a hairpiece look both better and worse. The answers were as follows.

Better

1. Not too much hair.
2. Hairline at an adult level, not a kid's hairline.
3. Hair color (less hair color contrast to the skin).
4. Permed or very curly hair.
5. No distinct hairline (like Robert Reed in "The Brady Brunch").

Worse

1. Too much hair.
2. Poor hair texture.
3. Hairline too low.
4. The frontal hairline and part.

Of all answers in my survey, it was the frontal hairline and part that was deemed the most obvious.

Hairpiece ads constantly hawk "natural hairlines" but in reality, the wearers are very unhappy with the effect. Bonded hairpieces will often lift after swimming or sweating anywhere from one day to four weeks after being glued on. No matter what attempts are made and no matter how good the hairpiece looks when the client leaves the facility where it was applied, patients tell me the next day is a whole new story.

Yet for some very bald or other appropriate patients, a hair system may be the appropriate choice in hair replacement. So how can it be made to look more natural?

In the past people (such as Ted Danson) who had hair loss behind the hairline would easily get away with wearing a partial hairpiece. I, myself, wore a partial clip-on hairpiece with virtually no detection (unless adverse circumstances occurred). The reason for this is the naturalness of the hairline. Sometimes I will have a potential patient come to talk with me and my secretaries will say they don't know why he's here, he seems to have a full head of hair. Invariably, when I see the patient, I too (but not as easily) can be fooled. The answer is always the same, his frontal hairline is his own. When asked why he's here, it's usually because of other problems he might have had with the hairpiece or the place that sold it to him.

One person told me the story of his going to the beach with a young lady whom he was getting along with quite well after several dates. His hairline was mostly his own, but his hairpiece (which was clipped on) was quite expensive. He didn't want to wear it, therefore, at the beach. When he parked in the lot, he opened his trunk, took out the blanket and cooler, and placed his hairpiece into a case. The girl had not known he wore a hairpiece because it looked so good with his natural hairline. He assumed the girl had liked him for himself at this point. Well, she never saw him again, telling him every excuse but what he perceived as the real one, that she was prejudiced against bald men. I told him perhaps he should have told her in advance that he wore a hairpiece rather then use "shock therapy." Would he expect her to be less shocked if he unscrewed a false leg at night before staying with her without giving some advanced warning?

This story helps deliver two points; not just America's love affair with appearance, but more importantly in this chapter, the undetectability of the hairpiece.

In an effort to make their hair systems more undetectable and thus more marketable, hair replacement firms have now been offering the combination approach—hairpiece plus transplant. With the newest technology turning out virtually undetectable growing hairlines, several organizations have now employed the advice and services of doctors skilled in transplanting the frontal hairline (I have performed several of these) and although the idea is not new, the technology of single hairs and small grafts, especially linear, allow the recreation of the natural feathering zone.

The way this is approached is by the patient first coming into the office with a temporary unformed hairpiece along with his hair replacement expert or hairdresser. The hairpiece is loosely placed one to two inches behind where the new hairline is to be created. Then, using marking pens, the new proposed hairline is drawn. The hairpiece is slid forward into this zone to ascertain the final look. If all seems acceptable to patient, doctor, and hair replacement expert, the hairpiece is removed and the patient is prepped for hair transplantation.

The conservative approach is important here; once again it is much easier to lower a hairline later on than to raise it if it's too low. This is advice only an experienced expert who has seen both knows.

It is also important post-transplant that nothing is glued to the fresh surgical site. These grafts are delicate and heal fast, but they can be damaged by tape or bonding. There are other means of safe camouflage, as I have mentioned, and they should be employed.

The result can usually be achieved in only one large session, but the patient should be made aware that a second procedure may be necessary to achieve his desired effect.

Patient selection is also important, as I would not wish to frontally transplant anyone who is not sure he will continue wearing a hairpiece or would consider other means of hair replacement in the future. *A procedure should not be performed on a patient just because he wants it to be done!*

In the properly selected and advised patient, however, the results can be terrific. People who would never have the hope of regaining a reasonable amount of hair with a natural look because of extensive hair loss (for various reasons) or poor donor area, can look like they never lost their hair. Patients also tell me that the hairpieces are more manageable because they don't have to spend hours covering the hairline. The systems are cheaper to make and easier to service as well.

Here, swimming and sports become easier with less chance of detectability because the hair is combed straight back, while wet, revealing a natural hairline with little chance of the hairpiece lifting behind it. This becomes especially true when the frontal hair is grown long enough to comb over the front of the hair system. When sweating, the hair of the piece will not get wet, but the frontal hair will and by combing it back over and integrating it with the hairpiece hair, it can look very normal as well. And here, if synthetic hair is used rather than human hair for the system, the piece will hold up much better in the sun. It will still need service, though, and you should not delude yourself into thinking that this is the perfect fix, just one far superior to the old hairpieces and systems.

EIGHT

WHAT IS A SCALP REDUCTION?

In layman's terms, a scalp reduction is a facelift to the back of the head. The back of the head refers in general to the bald or balding area on the top, middle, or crown regions.

The idea of scalp reduction was first published back in the 1970's by Drs. G. and B. Blanchard. The idea at that time was that a person had only limited available donor area available and thus it would be advantageous to shrink the amount of bald area to be covered. This would then allow the available donor area to be distributed over a much smaller bald area. Dr. Sparkul, also in the late 70's, realized that the scalp in many patients had extra "looseness" in the rear half. His theory was that if he performed a series of excisions of this extra tissue, he could slowly close the gap between growing hair. He further felt that if the surgeon didn't try to remove too much tissue at a single setting, he had a better chance for success.

In the late 70's and 80's, very few doctors closed the donor area (see donor closure). Because of this, plugs were removed from the donor sites and had to be spaced apart to allow for proper healing and coverage by adjacent hair, thereby making them undetectable. This significantly limited the available donor area. Transplant surgeons who tried to remove the hair plugs without leaving enough normal scalp between them often found a patient with scarred areas that would show, especially when the hair was wet. This very problem happened to me with my original transplants in the early 70's, and later had to be surgically repaired. Doctors, because of this complication, would rather have erred in taking the plugs further apart than necessary thereby "wasting" donor area than to risk the unhappy patient. This even further reduced the available good hair remaining for transplantation.

Also, hair transplantation to the crown of the scalp was never very successful unless the patient had permed hair. This was probably because hair laid differently in the crown and we could not simulate the original pattern very well. We were taught to direct the hair even in the crown in a uniform forward direction and this would make combing the hair to cover the "plug look" a virtual impossibility.

Back in 1976, one of my first patients approached me to finish a previous transplant. He had been Type V bald and, although his front two-thirds had grown well, his remaining bald area was obvious. When I checked his available donor area, I felt that he had little left to give. He then asked, "Can't you cut out some of the rest?" I had never thought about it and was reluctant to try (he was and still is a lawyer). After he prodded me repeatedly, I removed small areas of the part side of the remaining bald area, thereby lifting up the surrounding hair so he could comb it over to conceal what was still bare. His additional persuasive prodding convinced me to remove old scars in the donor area and to use the available hair between the scars to transplant additional areas and eliminate the suture line scar from the "reduction" (I didn't have a name for this in those years). This worked, but I was reluctant to try it on others for several years to come.

The 80's became the era of the scalp reduction, however, and by 1983 I had performed several hundred.

ARE ALL SCALP REDUCTIONS THE SAME?

In a word, no. Although the principal goal of all scalp reductions is to shrink the remaining bald area in the back top half of the scalp, surgeons began to disagree about how to accomplish this. The original scalp reductions were elementary and modelled after the method surgeons used to remove growths from skin. The best way to understand them is to categorize, criticize, and diagram them for you.

WHAT IS A MIDLINE SCALP REDUCTION?

This was the basic design. Here, an elliptical cut was made in the center of the bald scalp. The tissue within the ellipse was removed and the two edges were sewn together, pulling the hair-bearing scalp on both sides closer together.

This simple original operation would help eliminate as much bald skin as possible. The amount was determined by the elasticity (looseness) of the patient's scalp as well as the skill of the surgeon. In its simplest form it was logical and should easily work. The problems with it had yet to be discovered and are detailed later in this chapter.

After performing the first scalp reduction, surgeons felt (as per Dr. Sparkul's paper) that if we allowed enough time between procedures (anywhere from one to six months), the scalp would again loosen up and additional bald areas could be removed. In many cases this worked, in others it did not (see later). Patients who wanted a series of scalp reductions would often ask me if their ears would move to the top of their heads when they were finished. They wouldn't, so I used to smile and say "I hope not, but if they do, at least you'll hear approaching overhead aircrafts before the rest of us."

One of my favorite patients in this era was the son of the governor of a New England state. He told me that he would not begin a transplant to his frontal area until we got the back closed. Nine procedures over three years accomplished this, but this was an unusual case (he was Type VI) and fortunately had very elastic skin. This type of case, as many of us who performed scalp reductions were soon to find out, was rare enough to be a collector's item.

In order to prevent multiple scars on the top of the scalp, we would always include the previous scar as part of our next procedure. But this, the simplest and most basic of all reductions, would present too many failures and poor results, so many of us began varying the method in order to vary the result.

WHAT WERE THE PROBLEMS WITH MIDLINE REDUCTIONS?

The biggest problem with midline reductions was stretch-back, a problem that would also arise in many subsequent alternative methods. The original thought was that when you removed "x" amount of bald skin, there was that much less bald area left to cover. It became apparent, in follow up, that many patients still seemed to have bald areas after six to eight weeks that appeared no different in size from the original site. What was occurring was a stretching of the skin which caused four events.

1. The resultant gain of the original reduction might only retain 50 percent of the original amount achieved.
2. The scar site would widen.
3. The skin layer becomes thinner from stretching.
4. Slot defect—a wide and elongated center alleyway with poor or no hair growth and with surrounding hair growing downward away from the defect.

Stretchback was reported in a study by Dr. Nordstrom in the mid-eighties out of Norway where many more scalp reductions were being performed than in the United States. Reports of up to 50 percent stretchback were common.

Other problems were noticed later. In many cases of midline scalp reductions, the scar would indent creating what I nicknamed a buttocks deformity. This occurred because the suture line would be pulled in two directions and would, thereby, thin more than the surrounding scalp, creating an indented widened area.

A further problem of even very successful midline reductions was the hair angle. Since the sides were being evenly elevated, the hair which grows downward on the sides would be brought to the top of the scalp where the hair growth angle should face forward and not downward. Because it didn't, the hair became almost impossible to groom.

A series of multiple midline reductions on the same patient also thins the skin and decreased blood supply (scar tissue has less blood supply), causing a poorer take in the subsequent hair transplant grafts. What this all translated into was a good idea that had limited practical application. It's sad that many inexperienced doctors still choose this type of reduction because it is the simplest to perform. I stopped performing it back in 1984 and have published its pitfalls subsequently for other doctors to recognize.

I have seen in the past, several cases where the surgeon attempted to remove too much bald skin at one time. In these cases, it becomes very difficult to close the wound and even if you do, you can count on an ugly scar and poor subsequent transplant growth. I have seen one doctor actually put back some of the skin he removed to close the wound (yes, it retakes and is probably the smartest way to deal with this problem.) Others have just gotten the wound close together and let it heal by the formation of new scar tissue like a gash would heal.

No matter what the result or intention, one of the biggest problems with midline reductions is visibility. It's tough to cover a big scar dead center in a bald area, especially when the surrounding hair will not comb over it. I had one patient who came to see me because with his prior reduction result, he was nicknamed hatchet head. The scar was so straight and depressed that it really looked like he could have been hit by an axe. I corrected this by performing several small horizontal reductions through this vertical scar and subsequently slowly transplanted the area. Fortunately hatchet head's name returned to Steve F. and his life eventually returned to normal.

I am not saying that complications do not occur with any form of reduction surgery, but at least progress in this field has minimized them.

The final, and perhaps the most disfiguring result of midline scalp reductions is related to what's called the slot deformity. By taking out an elliptical central piece of bald scalp, one creates a suture line that is straight and longer than the curved edges of the ellipse. The result is a bald spot further toward the rear in the center of the remaining donor area, kind of a bald central pit.

This causes an abnormal appearance from the rear view and necessitates additional surgical correction.

Stay away from midline scalp reductions unless for an appropriate reason.

WHAT IS AN APPROPRIATE REASON TO HAVE A MIDLINE SCALP REDUCTION?

Midline reductions work well in nongenetic baldness where narrow small scarred areas from either burns, accidents, or even forcep delivery scars from birth are the target. Your experienced transplant surgeon should be able to advise you of what is appropriate and should allow you to talk to prior reduction patients to help you determine your decision. Make sure your surgeon performs many different types of scalp reductions and has extensive experience in each. I have seen many people, for example, who were advised by one transplant doctor not to have a reduction at all. Responsible colleagues who practice in the same area have told me that the reason this doctor never recommends a scalp reduction is because he has never performed one. You want objective advice, not advice targeted to the capabilities of the doctor.

WHAT IS THE MERCEDES STAR REDUCTION?

No, it is not a German luxury scalp reduction. In order to avoid the slot defect and to perhaps remove some additional bald tissue, doctors tried varying the midline reduction. They instead made a three-part reduction in the shape of the Mercedes star in order to decrease the bald area.

In theory, this reduction would seem to remove more tissue and help preserve hair growth angles a bit better than the midline variety, but in reality it had all the problems of the midline variety and now there were two slot deformities.

There were three hatchet chops and three areas for stretchback. In my opinion, this was a further disfiguring operation and even more difficult to correct.

You may like the car, but you'll hate the emblem on your head.

WHAT IS A LAZY S REDUCTION?

After it was noted that stretchback of up to 50 percent or more could occur, several of us felt that one of the reasons was based on a simple surgical principle: straight lines have equal and opposite forces pulling on them.

In an effort to combat this, surgeons began trying the lazy S reduction. This also served to eliminate the slot deformity because it would not go as far back on the scalp. The linear length of the cut, however, was equal to the older midline reduction because it curved in two directions.

This was the first attempt to avoid the opposite but equal tension forces because the suture line was curved and not straight.

The result of this was a significant decrease in stretchback. Additional procedures could be more successful as long as they incorporated the old scar.

Attempts to reverse the S shape on the next reduction proved to be disastrous in subsequent transplant procedures.

In addition, in the poorly chosen patient, these scars were still exposed in the center of the bald scalp and led to considerable embarrassment in the patient who had no camouflage. If later transplants grew poorly, disfigurement was a possibility.

WHAT IS A PARAMEDIAN REDUCTION?

In order to help hide the scar, surgeons began using a side incision (paramedian). This was closer to the existing hair and hooked like a "J" at the end in order to avoid the slot deformity. This, when performed on the part side, could help in coverage but it still had many of the pitfalls of the midline (median) reduction.

First it was mostly in a straight line and therefore had stretchback problems. Second, it brought the hair up on one side, but the hair angle was still wrong. This, as before, made it difficult to comb the hair over the remaining bald area.

But most important, it was also asymmetric. Hair was higher on one side than the other. The eye picks up this abnormality and focuses on it as it would a hairpiece turned sideways. Paramedian scalp reductions are rarely used now by the experienced transplant surgeon except in special cases. These are similar to the special cases for midline scalp reductions.

WHAT IS A CURVILINEAR (CIRCUMFERENTIAL) SCALP REDUCTION?

Back in 1986, after seeing the problems with prior scalp reductions performed by many experienced physicians including myself, I attempted to revise the format to avoid or help eliminate many of the problems seen in the prior scalp reduction varieties.

The curvilinear scalp reduction was the result of a patient's suggestion. Often, I have found, patients suggest ideas that make sense and I may, after trying them, subsequently incorporate them into my practice.

The curvilinear scalp reduction involves an incision curving along with the bald pattern. It almost looks like a smile on the back of the scalp.

By making the incision along the border of the bald area, I found that you could shrink the bald spot symmetrically, thereby preserving hair direction and angle. In other words, you could make a larger spot look like a smaller one. In some cases of good elasticity and a smaller size bald area, you could virtually eliminate the bald spot.

Another valuable result was that the patient could comb his hair properly helping to cover or disguise the surgical incision. Makeup or camouflage could be applied much more easily to an area near the existing hair eliminating the difficulties in covering the midline hatchet look.

Another advantage was that if the patient did not desire to complete a hair transplant in the crown, it was easier to disguise the scar by transplanting through it. This was because the scar was near the hair-bearing fringe and not in the middle of the head.

For several reasons, stretchback, the big menace to success in reductions, became less of an issue in the curvilinear (circumferential) procedure. One was that the laxity (looseness) of the scalp is most pronounced along the fringe hair borders in the back of the scalp. A second is that the stretchback vectors along the suture line which we discussed earlier are never in the same direction. Therefore there is no strong pull along the incision to enhance stretching.

To prove this, I undertook a study with a dermatologist in charge of the Hair and Nail Clinical Program at New York Hospital Cornell Medical Center. We took a series of over thirty patients and measured the amount of the reduction (distance between fringe hair). Measurements were taken before, immediately after, and both ten days and six months post curvilinear scalp reduction. We found and published in the *Journal of Dermatologic Surgery and Oncology* in 1989 both the technique of scalp reduction (''A New Technique for Curvilinear Scalp Reduction,'' October 1989) and the study results demonstrating that only 5 percent of cases experienced stretchback. These cases could then either undergo an additional reduction procedure or they could instead complete the area with hair transplantation. The beauty here was that once again, even if the patient did not want transplants in the crown (remember transplants didn't look all that great in the late 80's and early 90's) they could simply have the scar transplanted through and leave the rest of the area ''au natural.'' This, of course, could never be accomplished in scalp reductions involving the center of the scalp.

As our experience with circumferential reductions expanded, we started to see the half circle to ''U'' effect. What this meant was that the looseness of the scalp was far superior towards both sides than it was in the rear. This meant that we could remove a lot more bald skin safely from the sides than from the back of the scalp. The additional reductions would change the shape of the incision from a half circle to a "U." This would mildly distort hair angles and the experienced transplant surgeon knew to be more conservative in the amount of bald tissue removal to minimize this problem.

One of the other problems we saw with time was that in repeated reductions, subsequent hair transplantation graft growth was diminished when using the old round plugs. To help correct this, we would often transplant first in the rear center of the scalp and then reduce the surrounding area to closely meet it. This worked very well and there was no problem in later transplanting through the remaining fringe area.

Curvilinear (circumferential) scalp reductions are the present favorite of hair replacement surgeons. The advantages far outway the negatives, and though nothing is guaranteed, the negatives are far easier to correct. Even in the enhanced reductions incorporating extenders and expanders as well as in scalp lifting (all to be described later) the fringe curved incision has remained the most reliable surgical approach and has over time delivered the best results.

SO SHOULD EVERYONE HAVE A SCALP REDUCTION?

Many times I have had patients come to see me telling me to cut out the bald area in the back of the head. After examining them, I tell them that they have no bald area there. They then produce a picture of their father or uncle and tell me they never want to let themselves get to that point.

This contrasts with a favorite story of a well-known politician who came to see me and brought with him a videotape. He asked me to play it before we talked. On it was himself on national television addressing the American people and Congress. I thought that he was trying to either impress me or demonstrate his inflated ego until he suddenly paused the tape. He froze it at the point where he had turned around to talk to another political leader. At this point he ran to the T.V. and exclaimed, "Get rid of that bald spot, please." We subsequently reduced and later transplanted the area. His schedule of public appearances was so hectic that his case helped us develop further experience in the art of temporary camouflage.

Others have come in to the office with wedding, bar mitzvah, christening, or confirmation videos demonstrating a bald spot on the crown that they swear they never knew existed. All wanted immediate repair.

But today, with the type of donor harvesting and the new laser, single hair, micro and mini, and linear grafting techniques, we can resimulate the normal swirl pattern of growth in the crown. This has eliminated the need for scalp reduction in many candidates. The results with grafting alone have become superior to reduction followed by transplantation. Hair angles and growth patterns are more easily reestablished without the reduction first.

Nonetheless, in the very bald patient, circumferential scalp reductions are a valuable tool. Remember, you only have so much hair to donate, and therefore, in those with limited donor and maximum desire, a scalp reduction or two can be a big help.

I have two patients in mind, Alan R. and Richard L., who were both very bald. When they came to see me, at first they only wanted transplants to improve their frontal image. As time went on, they saw a good beginning and decided to shoot for the moon, but conservatively.

However, we first essentially completed the transplant to

the front of the scalp in order to make sure we had enough hair to refine our result and to give the patients time to be sure they really wanted to continue.

I met with both patients and their families, both together and separately, to help counsel them and answer any concerns and questions. It is important for your doctor to conduct a reevaluation during your procedure to help guide you through it since this is not a one-day event.

Alan R. had a loose scalp and we decided to utilize this to our best advantage. Because of the excellent healing and availability of additional donor area, I decided to perform a two-stage circumferential scalp reduction. I also decided to first transplant into the center of the remaining bald area to allow maximum circulation for healing and good growth. The linear grafts I transplanted were angled to recreate the swirl, and later with scalp reduction I hoped to bring his fringe hair very close to the transplanted area. After the transplants were well healed, I proceeded with the reductions. Following both reductions (six months apart to allow the best return of scalp elasticity), I was able to then transplant through the remaining bald area and mostly eliminate the suture line scar.

Comically, Alan came in one day showing me a traffic ticket he received for driving with someone else's license. He was laughing and proud that the police officer refused to believe he was the same person as the picture on his driver's license. Thus he was ticketed. I went to testify at his hearing and eventually wound up transplanting the police officer who had ticketed him.

Richard, on the other hand, did not have the looseness of Alan's scalp, but he did have one advantage; his head was narrow and long and, therefore, he had more donor area to give. I still performed a scalp reduction on him (every little bit helps) and then proceeded to finish the transplant. Although I might not choose to go this far with others, the results were remarkable.

One of the keys in deciding how far a doctor can go with any patient is the patient's patience and ability to work with a doctor over the long term. There is no quick fix here, and the doctor needs a patient who can both listen and hear. I could never have achieved what I did with Alan and Richard without their cooperation, patience, and dedication. I can't tell you how often I have had patients come to me with bald spots in the crown asking me to "cut them out." My response is invariable—"I'm not going to scalp you." If you want results, then understand that scalp reductions as well as transplants have their limitations and we have to work together through them.

So, as we have learned with so many medical procedures over the years, there is a time and place for most of them. The patient, his diagnosis, his prognosis, and his cooperation are key in answering the more specific question—Is a scalp reduction right for me?

WHAT'S AN EXPANDER?

We've discussed the basic scalp reduction. Now it's time to go one step further. In the past, in the case of accident victims who had scarred areas from injury, balloon-type devices were inserted under the injury to "stretch" the area and accomplish two goals. First, to free up the scarred area, and second, to expand (stretch) the skin and allow the added elasticity to facilitate closing the resulting defect (after excision).

This technique was first utilized in Scandinavia years ago. An expandable balloon-type device is placed under the skin and slowly inflated through an exposed valve. Daily, additional sterile fluid (sterile in case it bursts) is added to the balloon. After extensive inflating and a three-to six-month period of time, the skin is stretched enough to facilitate removing it and closing the remaining ends together. The reason that the stretching occurs over three to six months is to help destroy scalp elasticity and thus prevent stretchback of the resulting suture line.

When it came to a bald scalp, scalp expansion took on a new dimension. Doctors tried all sorts of expansion techniques and devices to accomplish this in an effort to maximize the amount of bald tissue to be removed. For our purposes, we will categorize the expansion into two categories—immediate and delayed.

Immediate Scalp Expansion

The original expansion was accomplished by inserting a small balloon-tipped tube (catheter) under the bald skin at the time of the scalp reduction. Here, the balloon is filled with as much fluid as possible during the surgery. It is left filled for several hours. At the end of this period, the scalp is deemed stretched and the extra tissue is removed. The two remaining tissue lines are then sewn together.

Delayed Scalp Expansion

Here the theory is that scalp elasticity takes time to defeat. Because of this, the patient has a balloon inserted under the bald area. This is slowly inflated daily with more and more sterile fluid. After several months, the scalp tissue is stretched permanently and the extra bald tissue is easily removed. Stretchback is minimized because the scalp is stretched out and no longer retains any remnants of its original elasticity.

WHAT ARE THE PITFALLS OF SCALP EXPANSION?

It sounds great. Stretch the bald area and then remove it. Well as you may have probably guessed, nothing comes for free. Here are the costs.

1. *Short-Term Expansion*
   Just like the midline scalp reduction, short-term intraoperative expansion lives up to its name—*short term.* Stretchback is a major concern here as stretching the skin is only temporary, and the skin will soon regain its elasticity. So the happy patient who thinks he's had a fabulous result may change his mind over the short period of time in which stretchback may occur. And the stretchback may be significant.

   In my opinion, scalp expansion of a short-term (intraoperative) basis can be gimmicky, and should mainly be used to *help close a difficult wound only.* I believe it's naive to think that a short term stretching of the scalp treats anything but the surgeon's ego. I have seen too many patients come in with stretched scars and deflated egos after short-term expansion. Always request to talk to the long-term patients of any short-term procedure to help you evaluate the results and appropriateness for your own situation.

2. *Long-Term Expansion*
   Here we have a better basis for a positive result. This is because it has been shown that the elasticity of the skin and the forces for stretchback will slowly decrease over time; in other words, the longer the period of time for which the skin is expanded, the less its ability to regain its original shape.

   A good way to think of this is compare it to buying a pair of shoes which are too narrow. The store will give them a quick stretch and they will, in general, feel better. But the next day, the tightness seems to return. This is especially true with leather shoes and remember, leather was another animal's skin once. The most effective way to get the desired stretching is by leaving an oversized wooden mold in the shoes for a prolonged period of time. This will defeat the resiliency of the leather.

   But shoes are not people, and long-term expansion has its complications. The most common of these is the deformity of a balloon under the skin. I call this the E.T. defect because it honestly makes the patient look like Spielberg's alien. As the expander is slowly inflated over a several-month period of time, the appearance worsens. Most of us do not have the luxury of being able to hibernate for three months instead of walking about, and certainly your career can be adversely affected by looking like the Elephant Man in public. Yet some brave the humiliation and embarrassment in their quest to "cure" baldness.

But if deformity of appearance was the only possible complication, then perhaps more men would brave this. The second complication, however, is pressure necrosis of the skin. What this means is that the constant pressure of a balloon stretching the skin will decrease the blood supply to it and can cause the overlying skin to die and slough off. If this occurs, the patient may have to undergo long-term skin grafting procedures and may wind up looking far worse in the end. In addition, the skin grafts will be thin, off color, and will probably never accept hair transplant grafts later on. One point to remember is that the patient has the balloon under his scalp. He is also not under the daily care of a physician who might detect early signs of decreased blood supply. Even if he were under the physician's care, the early signs may not prevent the eventual tissue slough.

Pressure bursting is another problem. The skin, like the inner tube of a tire, can accept only so much distension (tension). After this point, the skin, like the tube, may burst open to relieve this pressure. This is not a very welcome event in any case, but it is certainly a real possibility.

The stretching may cause other problems as well. The constant pressure may begin to cause pain and the pain can progress to unbearable levels. The pain may also be the first sign of skin ready to "burst" open. Also, by stretching and thereby thinning the skin, the remaining bald tissue may not accept transplanted hair very well and the resultant growth may be poor. This skin is generally shiny and the remaining bald area can therefore look peculiar.

Infection, of course, is another concern. Any foreign body inserted under the skin which has an outlet (valve) to the outside world opens a channel for bacteria to enter. Although infection here is rare, it can occur and in its worst form can require hospitalization, intravenous antibiotics, and the permanent removal of the device. Never take any insertion of a foreign body lightly. If you have the device inserted, you are responsible to help look for complications before they become problems. A good doctor will review along with you and give you the patient a list of the warning signs.

The final important downside of long-term expansion is hair direction. As I've mentioned earlier with midline scalp reductions, hair direction on the sides of the head grows downward, and hair on the top of the scalp grows forward. Since the balloons are removed with a midline cut, the same grooming problems related to midline reductions can happen here.

I'll probably repeat this statement several times—risk-taking is only worth the risk if the downside is correctable. If the downside may mean permanent odd bald areas or need for skin grafting to correct but not cure the problem, then the risk is probably not worth taking. Remember, even if the severe consequences occurs only once in a hundred cases (1 percent sounds low) and you are that one, the other ninety-nine successes will not make you feel that you did the right thing. The only person you will see in the mirror is yourself.

Scalp expansion is rarely performed in this country anymore for hereditary baldness with the exception of scalp flap procedures (see later chapter).

WHAT IS SCALP EXTENSION?

The problems and *especially* the deformity of scalp expansion helped give birth to newer ideas. In 1993, a French physician named Patrick Fretchet published an article showing impressive results with scalp extension. He would perform a midline scalp reduction, but at the same time insert an elastic strip with prongs on both ends. These prongs would clip on to the underlying tissue (galea) on one side, and then he would stretch the strip 100 percent and insert the prongs of the other end to tissue on the other side of the cut. This is the same idea as suspenders on pants.

The difference is that the stretch is considerable with the extender. The wound is then closed over it. The principle here is that over the course of several weeks, the extender will stretch the surrounding hair-bearing skin, creating a looseness to the bald skin between the hooks. This would then allow a second more extensive scalp reduction in which additional amounts of bald area, along with the device, could be removed. Dr. Frechet reported that even in "tight" scalps, his device could offer considerable help to a scalp reduction. In fact, Dr. Frechet claimed that he could improve the amount of tissue removed by over 50 percent. He further reported that he could perform a series of extensions to further reduce the bald area over time. I have seen some of these pictures (although not patients) and indeed the results appear impressive. But I have seen patients from other physicians, some in New York, where the results are not so impressive; in fact, they are downright ugly. Once again, when choosing your doctor, make sure he has extensive experience in performing what he suggests for you. I have seen doctors who have gone to watch Dr. Frechet at a conference or who visited him for a day in his office and who are now performing scalp extension. I wouldn't want to be one of their early patients.

Furthermore, Dr. Frechet has changed the type of reduction he performs to curvilinear (circumferential) to help avoid exaggerated versions of the complications of midline scalp reductions.

WHAT ARE THE COMPLICATIONS OF SCALP EXTENSION?

First, please bear in mind, as of this writing, scalp extenders have not been approved by the Food and Drug Administration. For this reason alone, I would not recommend this procedure.

A doctor in the U.S. may be able to insert this device, but that doesn't make it necessarily ethical to do so. Make sure you are informed before you have any procedure performed on you. This is not meant to scare you, however, as in the right hands and situation, scalp extension may be a great help in "curing" your bald condition.

That said, let me return to the question. The most severe complication of scalp extenders is staphylococcus aureus infection of the extender. In Dr. Frechets' reports, this is rare. I have heard of one patient in the U.S. (a plastic surgeon) who had this procedure performed on himself in California. He wound up with a severe enough infection warranting admission to an ICU (intensive care unit) in a hospital in New York. This infection is extreme, and most cases, I am told, can be treated by removing the device immediately along with oral or injected antibiotics.

A more annoying complication is a seroma, a tissue reaction to a foreign body that causes the buildup of tissue fluid. This fluid causes a noticeable swelling and is generally removed daily by needle at your doctor's office. This in no way, however, interferes with the result unless the fluid, during needle removal, becomes infected.

Almost all patients will experience some degree of seroma.

Pain is another complication of any surgical procedure. Dr. Frechet reported mild to severe pain mostly within the first day or so, especially when sleeping. Patients I've seen for second opinions in my office have told me the pain lasts longer, but I have not had the opportunity to interview patients of Dr. Frechet.

Delayed healing of the wound has also been reported in several cases. Here, the blood-tinged fluid (reaction to the foreign body) keeps draining through part of the wound site. This can occur for several weeks or until the device is removed.

An expected complication in all cases is slot formation. Here, as in midline reductions, the bringing of two edges of an elliptical incision together will push the back of the closure downward and will cause puckering of the skin. Dr. Frechet has devised a triple-flap procedure to correct this complication, but this is additional surgery.

Another noticeable problem is the decreased density of the remaining fringe hair. This becomes important when the person requires additional hair transplantation.

Remember, whatever the procedure, there can be a price to pay that is not necessarily monetary. Don't look at before and after photos and discount the between time. The road from here to there may and usually does have a few bumps. With the Frechet extender, you are committing yourself to multiple procedures and expense (the extender costs five hundred dollars alone). But as always, in the proper selected patient and with the proper selected physician, the result can be very gratifying.

HOW MUCH TIME IS THERE BETWEEN PROCEDURES?

Dr. Frechet recommends one month between procedures. This is probably the optimal time period for the scalp elasticity to be decreased enough to limit stretchback. His preliminary reports show limited stretchback. I believe this to be truth for him, but not so for others. Multiple procedures can be performed at one-month intervals as well.

SO SHOULD I HAVE A SCALP EXTENSION?

Maybe, maybe not. After reading the above, this is a decision you must weigh and make yourself. Remember, if your scalp is loose, you do not need extension. If you are not very bald in the back of the head you also do not need reduction or extension. I, as well as other experienced surgeons, can easily show you before and after pictures of impressive scalp reductions that remove every bit as much bald tissue as a scalp extension (see my before and after pictures of the lazy S and curvilinear reductions). Here the procedure is simpler, more cost effective, and requires less numbers of surgical procedures. There are other very bald patients with tight scalps where donor is limited and scalp extension may offer an advantage. In 1993, scalp extension offered an advantage that is not so important today. With the newer transplant grafting procedures like the single hair and linear grafts, and with the greatly improved donor harvesting which has given us more hair to utilize in the bald area than we ever thought possible, scalp reduction as well as scalp extension have become ancillary rather than primary procedures in most cases.

WHAT IS THE PROLENE OR PDS SLING?

John Patrick Schwinning M.D., F.A.C.S. is board certified in general and vascular surgery. He has performed literally thousands of difficult, detailed vascular operations. But in 1987, Dr. Schwinning was bald and personally miserable. He came to me as a patient and wound up a skilled partner.

In late 1994, Dr. Schwinning started applying his vascular experience to the art of scalp reduction surgery. He saw the pitfalls of stretchback and used his experience to address it. Although scalp extension was and is a very viable option, Dr. Schwinning chose to modify the curvilinear scalp reduction procedure to improve results and eliminate stretchback. His theory, presented to the International Society of Hair Restoration Surgery in 1995 and the American Academy of Cosmetic Surgery meeting in N.Y. in 1996, encompassed the knowledge that stretchback in scalp surgery can occur over a three-to six-month period. This being the case, he felt it was important to have some way of anchoring the skin to prevent it. His vascular surgery experience taught him that prolene (used in open heart surgery) could be placed at the base of the reduced area (galea) and connected to both sides post reduction to anchor the edges of the new suture line together and thereby prevent stretchback. He knew the suture had to remain in place for at least six months to allow for final healing. He also knew to free up the bald area as much as possible to maximize the amount of bald area reduced.

The result of all this was a quick modification of the curvilinear scalp reduction procedure yielding a predictable and stable result. Stretchback, measured in thirty-eight cases over a six-month to one-year period was 3 to 5 percent. Further results in over one hundred cases showed the results to be similar. The use of PDS came into play when one of my patients, a plastic surgeon, suggested it as an alternative to prolene. This suture dissolves after ninety to 120 days and the thought was, is it long enough? Further studies showed it to be the case and this has become the standard of our scalp reduction procedure.

WHAT ARE THE COMPLICATIONS OF PROLENE SLING SCALP REDUCTIONS?

The prolene sling scalp reduction does not alter the basic scalp reduction techniques I described before. The complications are the same as that of the primary procedure with a few additions.

Skin-Suture Spitting

I have seen a few cases of the PDS suture ends protruding through the skin before dissolving. This was probably a result of not cutting the ends of the knotted suture close enough. The treatment for this is to pull up on the protruding stitch and cut the end as short as possible. Once it falls below the skin edge, it will dissolve in time and not be a problem.

Suture Reactions

I have seen several cases of local skin reaction to the buried suture. This is handled by local treatment and has not become a long term problem especially after the suture dissolves. The key is to follow the patient and be sure healing is complete.

Depression Of Suture Line

All reductions can have this as a complication. Even in the best of procedures, the suture line may have some depressed areas. Prolene or PDS slings as well as normal reductions and reductions with scalp extensions may all have this. The key here is that we can transplant through the depression, both disguising and helping to eliminate it.

You, the patient, must be made aware that this is a possibility. Temporary camouflage is often used to hide it, but the patient must be cooperative and work with the doctor.

I recently had a patient who was on the prime time television news almost daily as a spokesman for the N.Y.C. Police Department. He knew that any procedure he had would be immediately focused upon. Yet, he had had prior poor transplants, was very bald (TYPE VI), and wanted to shrink the area in the crown around which he had had prior plugs. Reduction was the only way in my opinion since "extending" his well used prior donor area would have thinned it too much and would have been restricted by the prior scar tissue. He used invisible concealer the day after his reduction, making his procedure undetectable. Mild suture line depression was later transplanted through.

This case also points out the benefit of any reduction procedure having an incision near the existing fringe hair. This patient never could have had his transplant finished in the crown because of the amount of prior transplantation he had had plus the limited existing donor supply. As a result, I only needed to transplant through his scar thereby disguising it as well as eliminating some unsightly bald space between the twenty-five-year-old plugs and his remaining hair.

SO SHOULD I HAVE A PROLENE SLING REDUCTION?

You should not have anything unless you need it and the good outweighs the bad in both the short and long term.

If you are bald enough to need a reduction and your scalp is pliable, then a prolene sling reduction is a nice way to go. If the above is true but the scalp is tight, then you may wish to take advantage of an extender.

What I'm saying is, whatever the case, your treatment must be individualized. Make sure you talk to several experienced doctors (not sales people) and see if their opinions agree. If they don't, and if you still want a reduction type procedure to the crown, go with the one with the least complications and that is easiest to repair.

WHAT IS SCALP LIFTING?

Scalp lifting is a more complicated surgical scalp reduction that first appeared on the hair transplant scene in 1986. It was, in part, a solution devised by Dr. Dominick Brandy of the U.S. and Dr. Mario Marzola of Australia for the problem of stretchback in scalp reductions. It also addressed the limited amount of scalp shrinkage in patients with scalps that just didn't have great pliability.

Scalp lifting involves, an extensive surgical procedure where both the bald area and the remaining hair bearing areas are undermined (freed up from underlying tissue) and then slid closer together. Although this sounds like the typical scalp reduction, it is not. It is instead a much more complicated procedure that goes quite further.

The original scalp lifts involved cutting and tying off the ends of both occipital arteries. These are in the back of the scalp on all of us and act as the main source of blood for that area. The vessels are not very elastic and therefore restrict the distance that the scalp can be "lifted." Additionally, the scalp is freed up (lifted off the underlying tissue) down to the ears on both sides as well as to the nape of the neck in the back. This enabled somewhere between 30 and 60 percent additional lift, eliminating more of the bald area. The cuts were also longer, extending almost down to the sideburns in an attempt to close up some of the frontal baldness as well.

This procedure has been performed under various types of anesthetics from general to intravenous sedation. In the properly selected patients, the results can be quite dramatic.

And just as in scalp reductions, patients will still require hair transplantation to finish their result and to disguise the resultant scars derived from the surgery. Dr. Marzola no longer performs this procedure because of this.

ARE THERE ANY COMPLICATIONS?

As in all forms of surgery, the more complicated the operation, the more complicated the complications. Since scalp lifting is a form of scalp reduction, it will have all of those possible complications I have mentioned before, as well as a few more.

Stretchback

Stretchback is possible but less likely here because the scalp is freed so extensively that there is less tension on the suture line. But if too much tissue is removed or if the scalp is quite resilient, stretchback will once again become a factor.

Numbness of the Scalp

All surgery involves cutting, and cutting will temporarily cut the surface nerves that allow sensation. In most cases feeling will return in several weeks, but in some cases, partial loss of feeling can be permanent.

Scalp surgery is no different. Transplants and reductions will cause temporary numbness in most cases. Scalp lifting is an extensive procedure and as such will cause extensive numbness all over the scalp. This, in general, will reverse itself also.

Bleeding

More extensive and longer procedures can cut more blood vessels and can cause more blood loss. This is why it is so important to have an experienced surgeon with experienced assistants perform your procedure. The same procedure may be very simple in one patient and may prove to be very difficult in another. This is not always predictable in advance.

Good surgeons can make even difficult procedures look easy because they are prepared for all eventualities. But for a novice surgeon, blood loss in this more complicated procedure can become a problem. If you opt to have a scalp lift because it's appropriate for you, then have it done by someone who does a lot of them. Interview his assistants and ask them about their experience in helping the surgeon, as well as about how long they have been assisting him.

I had one patient who came to me with a past scar from a "scalp lifting" procedure. I don't believe that's the procedure he had based on the location of the scar, but that's what he was told he had. I then asked him about the surgery. He told me that the doctor had no assistants and he was asked to bring his wife along in case the doctor needed help. In return for this, his price was reduced. The doctor explained to the patient that he had two assistants normally, but one had quit and the other had called in sick. The patient went ahead with the procedure anyway. The wife was asked to hold pressure and help stop the bleeding but she passed out (the sight of blood can do that to many of us). The result was the patient was transported to the hospital to stop the bleeding and wound up on iron pills to help replenish his red blood cells.

So is bleeding a problem in this more complicated surgery? Yes, if you are in the wrong hands.

Another possible complication relating to bleeding is a hematoma. A hematoma is a collection of blood under the surface of the skin. In its simplest form, it is what we call a black and blue mark. The color and swelling is partly from broken blood vessels under the skin and some resulting bleeding and blood collection. In general, the fact that our skin is bound to the tissue underneath will limit the bleeding and resulting hematoma. But in scalp lifting, the skin is freed up extensively and postoperative bleeding can become a problem. Good compression dressings and instructions from your doctor will limit this problem. But you, the patient, must listen.

I had a patient who is a fifth-degree black belt in martial arts who had an extensive scalp procedure. He was told to go home and rest. At 1:40 a.m., he called me to say that he was bleeding. I asked him to exert pressure on the area and come meet me in the office (he had someone to drive him). By the time he had gotten to the office, the bleeding had stopped, but he, at first, was quite evasive about what happened. His bandage was off and some stitches had ripped through one edge of the skin. Honestly, he looked like he was mugged. Finally, in private (his girlfriend was the driver) he told me the circumstances. From the office he stopped at the gym to work out and then sparred with one of his martial arts students. He reported receiving only a few kicks in the head. From there he went to see a girlfriend with whom he had an intimate two hours. But his day was not over. He then went to see his ''other'' girlfriend (the one who drove him) and they proceeded to have wild sex, during which she stuck her fingernails accidentally through his incision. At this point he decided to call me to report the bleeding. Needless to say, I was not pleased at the hour or the circumstances surrounding his episode. As a patient, you have to follow your doctor's instructions no matter how invincible you think you are. I had to redo his suture line and no problem resulted, but the whole escapade was not macho, it was dumb.

Permanent Hair Loss

One of the most important and devastating complications of the earlier scalp lifts was permanent thinning or loss of hair in the previous donor area. This was because cutting both occipital arteries interrupted most of the blood flow to the follicles in the previously good donor area. What's worse is that this is permanent and disfiguring. It just is not normal to lose hair in the lower half of the back of the scalp. I have seen several patients with this complication and the only remedy you can offer them is a full stretch wig. This is because you have to cover an area that wigs in general don't cover. Others have tried hair extensions, but the remaining hair proved fragile and the extensions would rip off easily.

Scalp lifting has improved since then and doctors now performing them are more careful about interrupting the blood supply. Classically, the patient will have the arteries tied off before the procedure to allow another blood supply to develop before the surgery. This has significantly reduced this devastating complication.

Scarring

As in scalp reductions, the scar can either expand or depress. But once again, because scalp lifting is conducted along the fringe hair, it becomes much easier to disguise and eventually transplant through.

SO SHOULD I HAVE A SCALP LIFT?

As in all other areas of hair replacement surgery, you must determine if this is a procedure for you. The newer modifications of scalp reductions as well as the vast improvements in hair transplantation really do reduce the need for this more drastic procedure. I always tell patients to look at the down side. By this I mean that if there is even a small chance of a devastating complication and it happens to you, then you are not going to care about the other 99 percent to whom no bad aftereffect occurred. You are going to care about remedying the problem. This is why if you can stick to more conservative measures, even if a complication exists, it can be more easily dealt with.

Nevertheless, the experienced surgeon should help you decide what procedure is right for you and in the properly selected, very bald patient, a scalp lift may be just the right medicine. As always, review your options with several doctors and be sure your chosen doctor is proficient in all different types of procedures. You don't want a physician who recommends the same specific procedure to all of his patients because this is what he exclusively performs.

And if your doctor is *bald*, ask him why. I am writing this portion of this book while attending a conference sponsored by the American Academy of Cosmetic Surgery. It seems that there is an abundance of bald hair transplant physicians here discussing the various treatments including scalp lifting. I asked several of them why they don't have the procedure or any other hair replacement surgery. The answers ranged from ''I have poor donor'' to ''Mind your own business'' and ''It doesn't bother me.'' Well, I still liken it to going to a weight reduction doctor who is a hundred pounds overweight. He may not care, but I do.

NINE

WHAT ARE SCALP FLAPS?

In simple terms, scalp flaps are an attempt to get naturally thick immediate growing hair to cover key parts of a bald scalp. Their history goes back to the mid 1970's when an Argentinian physician, Dr. Juri, published a paper describing the use of a skin flap to replace bald tissue. What he described and, in general, what flaps entail, is a major surgical procedure requiring general anesthesia where an attached piece of hair-bearing skin is freed up from the underlying tissue and is then rotated to the top of a bald scalp. To do this, a bald strip of skin must first be removed. The flap is then rotated into the prepared area and sewn in place. Blood supply is maintained by keeping the base of the flap attached in its original site. (See insert photos 14–15.)

After waiting several weeks to allow new blood supply to form for the freshly positioned skin, the base is then detached in a second operation and the flap is complete.

By not interrupting blood supply, the hair, in theory, will continue to grow and there will be no shock phase.

Now, mind you, this is very different than advancement flaps (such as what some have called scalp reductions) because we are actually freeing up a "tongue" of skin from the sides of the hair-bearing scalp and then twisting them carefully to fit on the top of the head.

In the latest and probably most popular procedure involving flap surgery, the initial phase involves the insertion of a balloon (scalp expander) under the scalp in the area in which the flap is to be taken. This is gradually expanded over several weeks until the skin is deemed stretched enough to be able to rotate a flap and still close the primary wound (the skin edges around which the flap was removed). Following this, in the next phase, the flap is lifted and rotated to its new home on top of the scalp. In the third and final phase, the last remaining connection of the flap to its old home is severed and any remaining deformities from the surgery are corrected. This is a multiple-staged and somewhat complicated procedure involving both doctor and patient cooperation to help insure its success. The flap, in this procedure, can be wider (1½ to 2 inches) because the expander has stretched the scalp enough to allow more skin to be removed and still allow the primary wound to be successfully closed.

The lure of the flap, in theory, is the immediate growth of hair. In some, this can be a strong lure but remember my old persistent piece of advice—be careful of the correctability of any potential complications.

At the time of this writing, I am taking care of a patient who flew to California from New Jersey to have a flap procedure. He was bald in the temporal regions (triangles) in the front only. He underwent two flap procedures (one for each side) and about six corrective ones. The problem was that part of the flap on one side became infected and necrosed (died), leaving an unsightly situation. Furthermore, the created hairline was too low and straight giving the appearance of a bad wig. He was forced to comb his remaining hair forward in a Caesar comb in order to cover the new bald spot and the abnormal hairline. In addition, unfortunately, he developed wide scars in the area from which the flap was taken. He now has spent upwards of forty thousand dollars and is miserable.

When I first met this patient, he was still flying back to California for his corrective surgery. His biggest and most memorable comment was, "If I only knew what I was getting myself into, I never would have even started." After waiting six months for proper healing, I performed one session of single hairs along the harsh flap hairline and small linear grafts within the areas the flap that did not take. The result was a cosmetic improvement so when the wind blows he no longer looks like Eddie Munster. Further work is needed, but I will work at the patient's pace. He's just happy he no longer looks freaky and is simply tired of surgery. Fortunately he owns his own large business and therefore was able to take the extensive time off from work that he needed to deal with the surgery and its complications.

HOW DID THE IDEA OF FLAPS DEVELOP?

For many years, surgeons have used the concept of flaps to cover large injuries such as from accidents or burns, or for skin cancer. It was not uncommon for a surgeon to use the skin's own natural stretching as well as areas of excessive skin such as the face, neck, and scalp to help cover surrounding areas destroyed by injury or surgery. Doctors learned early on that by keeping a wide base to the tongue-shaped, full-thickness strip of skin that was to be moved, there would be no interruption in the blood supply. The healing and cosmetic effect was also seen to be far superior to the old "split thickness" skin grafts where only a surface layer of thin skin would help hide a defect. In the old case the skin would be off color and depressed. The cosmetic effect is thus disfiguring when used in the wrong location. The full thickness flap would heal with normal color and thickness of skin in general.

These needs led to the development of creative ways to move the surrounding skin to cosmetically cover the newly created problem. We see this especially in facial surgery where skin cancers or other suspicious lesions are removed.

If the techniques worked on other parts of the body, it made sense that they could be modified to work on the scalp. Why not use the excess scalp tissue to rotate to bald areas (think of baldness as a bare lesion)? The idea was intelligent and thoughtful. The results, in my opinion, are far less.

WHAT KINDS OF FLAPS ARE THERE?

Flaps can be broken down into two categories—advancement and free. The advancement flaps as I mentioned are more like aggressive scalp reductions and fit into the previous category of scalp lifting. The free flaps fall into various categories according to their size and shape—for example, there is the short flap, BAT flap, TAT flap, and even the vertical flap.

WILL FLAPS COVER MY WHOLE BALD AREA?

In general terms—*no*! Flaps have certain limitations. For example, the maximum width of most flaps is only an inch.

Also, the thinner the base (the blood supply comes in here), the shorter the flap must be. Think of it as a tree whose trunk must enlarge for the tree to grow in order to get necessary nutrients to the top branches.

Now the scalp is looser on the top than the sides and remember, if you cut out a strip of scalp, you have to close both sides. An inch can be a lot for one to close well cosmetically. As a result, the number of flaps you can have performed on your scalp is limited, maybe three at most, and three flaps of even an inch width will not go very far. As a result, if flap surgery is your route, you will in all likelihood need additional procedures, even if the flaps take perfectly. Refinement of frontal hairlines is almost the rule in flap surgery and this usually requires micro and single-hair grafting. Spacing between the flaps will also call for subsequent reductions and/or hair transplantation. Additional hair loss later in life can cause additional problems, so flaps may not be appropriate in the younger patient with hair loss.

CAN A FREE FLAP HELP ME?

In some cases, it probably can. In the person, for example, with an injury or burn damaging a piece of scalp (which might prevent hair transplantation) or the person with very kinky or curly hair, the flap can provide a quicker cosmetic resolution for baldness. Most of us involved in hair replacement surgery, however, feel the role of the flap is diminishing as the safer and less extreme procedures of hair transplantation and scalp reductions have developed. Successful flaps compared to old big plugs were light years ahead. They provided thicker and more consistent hair growth without the old corn row effect. But today, the new techniques are quicker and look very natural. So why put yourself through expensive major surgery with possible considerable complications when today your options are so much more diverse?

There are those patients, however, who want areas of natural thickness especially towards the front of the scalp. In this, no procedure provides thicker coverage than a successful flap, but remember, *successful* is the key word. I have seen flaps on a patient performed in Japan twenty years ago. One side took, one side didn't. The side that took looked great and this patient used it to comb over a hairpiece to cover the rest of his bald area. The other side healed well enough to transplant through. For some reason, it had only a few hairs. The doctor was not to blame, either. The patient told me that his surgeon had performed thousands of flaps, and indeed his doctor's surgical precision was evident here. His procedure was not so radical as to make this patient uncorrectable. Still, the procedure failed.

As always, every patient is different and has different concerns and needs. Multiple consultations and good reference reading can help you make your proper choice.

WHAT ARE THE DANGERS OF SCALP FLAPS?

First it is major surgery requiring general anesthesia. This, in itself, can be risky, especially when it is for vanity and therefore not necessary surgery. And remember, the more major the procedure, the more major the potential complications. But to answer your questions, let me categorize and explain the potential complications.

Poor Growth

Here, as in hair transplantation, good surgical skill is the first and foremost necessity for a good result. But poor growth can happen in flap surgery even with a well-executed procedure. The possible reasons for this are interruption of blood supply to the flap causing hair follicles to die even if the skin of the flap survives. Also, too narrow a base will prevent the far end of the flap from receiving enough nutrients for the hair to survive and grow. Over twisting of the flap can similarly decrease blood supply with the same result. Another cause may be poor surgical technique in the removal of the flaps, which thereby injures the hair roots.

Flap Necrosis

In this case, blood flow is either cut off completely or restricted so severely as to ''kill'' not only the hair roots but the skin as well. This was true in the case I mentioned earlier where parts of the flap actually turned black and needed replacement. Flaps may also die from the balloon expander, exerting too much pressure. The over stretching will press against the potential flap with enough pressure to prevent blood flow from reaching all parts of the skin. Flap death is unsightly and in extreme cases, may not be fully correctable.

Pain

This is a common complaint when the expander is used. I had a patient today (quite coincidentally) who came to see me with a flap in front. It looked reasonably good, although the hairline was a bit low. The patient had had a previous single-hair megasession before deciding on the flap as his next remedy. He was unimpressed with the lack of hair density and believed flap surgery would be his answer. The patient came with his mom who was very bitter and suspicious about any further treatments. I asked both why, as his flap had fully taken and he looked, for his stage, fine. The answer took forty-five minutes, but I will give you the short version.

It seemed that the megasession had cost him over ten thousand dollars of his hard-earned money (he is twenty-six). When it failed, he borrowed over twenty-five thousand dollars from his parents for the flap surgery plus airfare and hotel costs to California. He flew there and came back with an expander under his scalp. He explained the pain was so constant and severe that he stopped going to work and flew back and forth to California to ask for it to be removed. He was talked into keeping it, but the pain got worse. No local physician was comfortable treating him, so he and his parents flew back to California and demanded its removal. Once again they were told he went through the worst of it and was talked into staying in California. He took a leave of absence from his job (without pay) and saw the procedure through. He now has his flap in place along with almost complete numbness and parastheslas (weird sensations) to the whole left side of his head where the flap has come from. He said he still had nightmares from the experience and would never consider a second flap as was recommended to him. My suggestion was to simply use larger transplant grafts behind his flap to finish thickening the top and place single hairs in front to soften the hairline. He is young, and with the low flap placement, one has to hope he doesn't go extremely bald.

P.S. He was also upset his flap doctor was bald.

Hair Direction

Hair normally grows in a forward direction in the front half of the scalp. This is standard in all Caucasians but not all Afro-Americans. Flaps can only be rotated in a certain direction to reach the top of the scalp. Because of this, the hair direction which goes downward on the sides of the head will now be redirected to grow towards the crown.

This will limit your hair styles depending on quality and type of hair. For example, African-American hair grows perpendicular to the scalp surface and therefore hair direction will not be a problem in those with kinky or permed hair. Hair direction is similarly of no consequence because the hair is coiled and will naturally mesh. It will also fall over the new hairline and can easily disguise a multitude of problems.

Hair direction becomes a much more important consideration when you have straight dark hair on light skin. Here, the hair is normally directed forward offering the ability to comb the hair to one side, part it in the middle, or even comb it forward in a Caesar (or Paul Simon) look. The flap hair will be directed toward the rear mostly preventing the ability to comb the hair over the new hairline.

Hair styles become limited, and unless one is very creative, the hairline will show and be obvious. Also, because the area behind the front flap generally remains bald, one may need further transplant work or need to comb the hair to cover the naked spots behind the hair bearing area.

You never realize how important hair direction is until you no longer have the proper one. This is why many patients with prior flaps, even successful ones, will come to see me complaining that people think they are wearing a hairpiece. Odd hairstyles draw attention to the hair just as parting the hair by the ear and then combing it over the top of the head will do. Both may disguise a bald area, but both are very obvious in their own way.

This then will restrict the patients' options. Most are told to perm their hair afterwards in an attempt to ease the time necessary to look presentable when getting ready for a day out or at work.

What I have done in these cases is to simply place single hairs and small linear grafts in front of the new hairline so as to make the direction of the hair less obvious and therefore important. Once the eye sees a soft transition of hair growing in the proper direction, it will no longer focus on the problem area behind it.

In my experience, I have seen several patients who presented to me not with hair loss, but with crazy cowlicks that they were just tired of dealing with. I remember one patient in particular who had a shock of white hair growing backwards right at the front center of his hairline. He said people thought that he had purposely bleached the hair white and believed he was a member of some cult or rock group. He wanted me to remove the white lock of hair and replace it with normal growing hair from the back of his head. I performed this relatively simple procedure and made one happy patient out of him. Let me also point out that it wasn't only the hair color that bothered him. When I first suggested he dye the white lock black (his hair color) he showed me pictures of himself with this accomplished. He still hated the wrong hair direction. To convince myself that it was right to do this transplant (after all he was not bald), I sprayed temporary color on his white hair. Although it was clear that the color was no longer a problem, it was very clear that hair direction still was. Seeing this, I didn't have any qualms about going on to perform his procedure.

A second case comes to mind in which a young man and

his father came to see me. The boy had his hat on and refused to remove it until I locked the door to my office. When he removed his hat, it was obvious to me that he had had a previous flap. His hair growth was thick, but his hairline was like Dracula's and his hair direction was straight back. He had very fine and very straight black hair and no matter how you tried to comb it, it would reassume it's slicked-back look. He had gone for a perm, but has hair was such that it would not last for more than one to two weeks. His scalp had also reacted to the perm chemicals and thus he had to stop any further permanent waves. His father was a combination of tears and anger and notified me that he was suing the boy's surgeon. The boy just turned to his father and stated, "But how does that help me?"

Here I was stumped. The hairline was far too low to disguise by lowering it further, even with single hairs. Electrolysis wouldn't work because the flap was slightly elevated and off color, so removing hair would only make it look worse. In addition, he had scars on the sides of his head from his flaps and he was forced to "tattoo them" to help prevent them from showing through his side hair. I referred this patient to a good plastic surgeon, Dr. Alan Engler, and together we began a program of scalp reductions higher up in an attempt to lift the hairline and shape it properly in the corners. After achieving as much as we possibly could, Dr. Engler performed some endoscopic brow lift surgery to further raise the forehead and with it, the hairline. Finally, we performed a re-transplant, where we actually thinned out this thick black-haired flap especially in the frontal zone to create a more natural see-through front. We then added a zone of single hairs in the proper direction in front of the hairline. Finally, we transplanted through his front flap in a very unusual fashion. What I did was to take out strips of hair from the flap and turn them around. In other words I used the flap as both the donor and recipient area. I removed my linear strips of hair and retransplanted them to the same site but now in the proper direction. Several properly spaced sessions of this turned out quite a respectable result. I must say that the creativity I had learned in my surgical training along with the skill and excellent eye of Dr. Engler helped me to help this twenty-one-year-old.

Others have not been as lucky.

Scarring

Scarring can occur in two areas. Historically, scarring has always been focused on the recipient site. In other words, if the flap doesn't take well, the scar can be downright ugly. But we will also focus on the donor area. A large scar in an area not easily covered by the surrounding hair or by a hairpiece can be devastating.

One of my patients brought me a videotape of a program his girlfriend had watched on NBC T.V. Here they talked about a patient who had had eleven flap procedures. The first three were an attempt to cover his bald area, and the last eight were attempts at correction. I don't often cringe, but this patient had giant scarred bald spots all over his scalp. Scars were in the lower neck region as well as higher up and thus hairpieces could only partially cover the problem. It was lucky I had transplanted his cousin several years back, because without his cousin bringing him in physically, this patient would have again chosen a glued on hairpiece even though he had previously thrown one away.

As I have said before, and will continue to repeat for those of you who might miss it elsewhere, choose a procedure where if you have a complication it is correctable and not devastating.

SO SHOULD I HAVE A FLAP?

As long as you understand the possible benefits and consequences of any procedure, you can make that decision. You must be prepared to have time off from work and you should stay locally during the procedure in order to have the doctor available to care for any problems.

I think flaps made more sense a few years ago. Today, with the vast improvements in hair transplantation and scalp reduction surgery, a flap becomes an unnecessary procedure. It's easy to be lured by the thought of immediate growth and thick hair, but as in the case of a hairpiece, unless the work is excellent a thick result can look worse than being bald. The difference between the two, however, is that you can remove a hairpiece and start over. In flaps, this is not a viable option.

At a recent conference, I was talking with several of my colleagues about their experience with patients and flaps. Most of them agreed with me that flaps will soon become a part of the history and no longer the forefront of hair replacement surgery.

WHAT ABOUT THE COST?

Flap surgery is probably the most costly of all surgical hair replacements. Flap prices range from ten to twenty thousand dollars each and these prices often do not include the cost of anesthesia and operating rooms. They also certainly do not include the costs of travel (if your doctor is not local) as well as hotel expenses. But most importantly, it does not include the loss of income for the time spent away from your work unless yours is a field in which you can have others substitute for you without loss of income, unless you own your own business or work from home. The balloon deformity is not a desirable conversation piece in the workplace.

So to tally the costs, we are talking about figures that can add up to sixty to over one hundred thousand dollars. If flaps are your route, you must be prepared for the bumpy road through it.

TEN

WHAT ARE THE COSTS OF HAIR TREATMENTS, REPLACEMENTS, AND SURGERY? HOW DO THEY COMPARE?

I had a patient who knew I was writing this book. He recommended that I include this chapter because, as he had gone through a myriad of different hair replacement avenues, he never realized what some of these could cost. He was age forty, and his post-transplant estimate was that if he lived for another thirty years, the hair would cost him twelve cents per day. Not all of us will go to this extent of analysis, but in some cases, when approaching your hair loss problem and how to solve it, it's not a bad idea. In writing this chapter I thought of what I spent over twenty years ago to cure my problem. When I added up the figures, I was astounded to realize that it cost me upwards of fifteen thousand late 1960's and early 1970's dollars. Today that would translate to nearly fifty thousand bucks. I also realized that if I had the proper guidance, my cost would only have been a fraction of that figure.

Hair replacements, both surgical and nonsurgical, can become expensive over time. Here are a range of costs for the various types of procedures.

HOW MUCH WILL MINOXIDIL COST?

Rogaine, Upjohn company's brand name of minoxidil, costs about fifty-five to eighty dollars per month, depending on your pharmacy. This, however, does not include the charges for office visits to see your doctor. These can range from one hundred and fifty to three hundred dollars per visit, not including any lab testing your doctor deems necessary. Doctors visits are generally scheduled four times per year. This will add up to approximately sixteen hundred to two thousand dollars annually. Now if you use minoxidil with Retin A or other ''special'' ingredients, the cost for medicine per month can go as high as ninety-five to one hundred and fifty dollars monthly, increasing your annual costs to over twenty-five hundred dollars!

Minoxidil (Rogaine) is now available over the counter. This has decreased the cost to about four hundred dollars a year. But this is still without the guidance of a physician, which can be a serious mistake.

CAN I KEEP THE COST LOWER?

Yes. There are several ways to save money and still be on the right dosage of Rogaine. One way is to buy the economical, now over-the-counter, triple packs (three-month supply) which reduce costs to approximately twenty-five dollars per month. Second, you can combine a vacation with savings by going to a Caribbean island such as Santo Domingo where the same quality product sells for less than twelve dollars per bottle. There is no U.S. customs restriction, as far as I know, to bringing an F.D.A.-approved medication into this country. Always check first as regulations can change.

You can also look for a physician who charges very little for followup Rogaine visits if you are smart enough to avail yourself of these. Many doctors will reduce fees for the brief and simple followups for patients on minoxidil. Remember, minoxidil taken internally is a dangerous drug. Just because it's over the counter now won't prevent you from accidentally overdosing.

For those using the ''special'' products, you can save in two ways. First, you can negotiate with your doctor for a reduction in the cost of the product. I have seen many patients from the same doctors pay varying amounts for the same product. Buying in volume if you plan to use it for several months will also save you money.

If you still feel that the price is too high, ask for a prescription for the doctor's ''special medication'' and then shop out pharmacies to receive the lowest price. Often you will be surprised to find that the cost from a responsible pharmacist can be far less than buying the ''special medication'' through your physician's office.

WHAT WILL AN EXOTIC FORMULA OR CURE COST?

I recently shopped the catalogs and mail order to get an idea of the range of price for the various over-the-counter cures for hair loss. What I discovered was that the cost can be higher than that for Rogaine. Add to this the fact that they don't work, and like myself in my early attempts at solving my hair loss, you have a big expense. Also most of the people incurring this expense are young and therefore least able to afford it.

A review of several self-help-type catalogs discovered products that ranged from starting kits for two hundred to three hundred and fifty dollars, to shampoos, conditioners, and capsules of miracle oils selling for about eighty dollars for a one-month supply. Now if you add in the vitamins which "target" your hair loss as well as the special tool to stimulate your scalp's blood flow, you are approaching one hundred dollars per month for nothing. It's no wonder that when the Helsinki formula was brought to court, it was revealed that the owners had made hundreds of millions of dollars.

WHAT DO HORMONE INJECTIONS OR DROPS COST?

Although most of us no longer inject the scalp afflicted by male pattern hair loss with cortisone or rub the scalp with progesterone or antitestosterone drops, these treatments still exist. Some swear by them although I have not personally seen any hair loss reversal or slowing as a result of their application. They are probably more suited for non-hereditary hair loss such as in alopecia areata.

When I tried the above cure as a balding young man, I was charged sixty dollars per month. When I asked the doctor why it was so expensive (remember this was 1970), his answer was that the cortisone and/or antitestosterones such as progesterone were extremely expensive. He went on to tell me that he was doing a study on these chemical treatments and was only charging me what it cost him. Years later I discovered that the cortisone as well as the other medicines cost only pennies. They could have cost nothing for the value they served me. My cost over two years was about fifteen hundred dollars (including special shampoos). The cost today is probably a bit more because of the added expense of lab tests and medical office visits. So if you wish to explore this route, expect to spend about one thousand dollars per year.

HOW MUCH WILL A PERMANENTLY ATTACHED HAIRPIECE COST?

The range of prices for all hairpieces are as diverse as the range of price for all cars. There is cheap and there is expensive. And as in many aspects of life, you don't always get what you pay for.

Hairpieces range from twenty dollars to over two thousand dollars. The twenty-dollar varieties are usually costume quality stretch wigs that fit over your head like a shower cap. Their bases are generally thick and wearing them for any period of time is almost impossible. You could no more wear this than the shower cap all day long.

Most good self-applied hairpieces cost in the neighborhood of five hundred dollars. Here you have purchased a light see-through-based piece with either synthetic or human hair. Most people will purchase two or three pieces at a time to limit the wear on each piece and to allow servicing to one, which costs about eighty dollars, while wearing another wig. Expect to have the hair dyed at least twice yearly (sixty dollars) and to have additional hair that is lost during normal wear replaced twice yearly as well (eighty to one hundred and twenty dollars). Single hairpieces will need replacement between eight months to two years depending on the level of care you give plus the environment you expose it to. If you are an outdoor person or live in a sunny climate, you can expect to replace the hairpiece after eight months. Supplies to attach the piece are not very expensive but you would be wise to purchase them at a beauty supply wholesaler where double-stick tape will cost only a few dollars for a large supply. You do not need special shampoos so don't be tricked into buying expensive ones.

Total cost per year for the above program—twelve to fifteen hundred dollars.

Now if you are really into undetectability, you may opt for a lace-front hairpiece. Here, the delicate lace mesh has individual strands of hair tied to the front and with the application of some camouflage or makeup, these hairpieces can look very good. The cost factor, however, can be up to two thousand dollars for a good one, and the repair record and cost is atrocious. If you opt for this route, expect to spend at least twenty five hundred dollars yearly. Your start-up cost will also be high because you will require a minimum of two hairpieces—cost about four thousand dollars.

WHAT SHOULD HAIR SYSTEMS COST ME?

In the pages of the *New York Post* once every week, I see an advertisement entitled "Don't be scammed." The ad refers to the cost of hair systems—both the price of the system itself and the monthly cost of maintenance. The ad goes on to claim that the price for systems and ongoing repair are very often dependent on one's ability to pay and are not necessarily related to quality. This I have definitely observed to be true. I have had patients come into the office with the most godawful-looking system that upon questioning I discover is only six months old. When I ask the price they paid, it is not unusual to hear quotes between twenty-two hundred and four thousand dollars. I have similarly seen units that look pretty good, that are older, and that the cost was about twelve hundred dollars.

Not too long ago while assisting CBS T.V. news in a story about hairpieces and systems, I was able to talk to and visit some of the suppliers to the industry. What amazed me (and the consumer reporter) was that the cost of a typical unit supplied to these big chain hair system places averaged forty dollars. I was further told that the hair was "commercial" and dyed to easily match the sample for the client submitted. So the question arises, why should they cost several thousand dollars? The answer was, "Because they can get it."

So what should all of this cost you, the consumer, if this is the route you choose to take?

Well, according to the American Hair Loss Council and several independent hair salon professionals (such as Donte from For Men Only in Queens, N.Y.), a truly custom-made unit with good-quality hair should cost you between twelve to fifteen hundred dollars. It should last for one and a half to two years and should not fade as readily as the commercial units. You will need at least two units (one unit can be embarrassing if there is a problem with it). For example, I had one patient whose unit had loosened and blew off and out a car window—now he was stuck waiting for a substitute. This is a start-up cost of about twenty-five hundred to three thousand dollars. You will do better if you make a deal for two to begin with. Never be afraid to bargain price. Bring in competitors' advertisements and ask, if their price is cheaper, why.

A favorite trick I pass on during consultations is to have the potential hair system client visit the salon's waiting room without an appointment. Don't be afraid to ask prices—clients love to discuss it amongst themselves. Also question prior clients on the price of service and any extra charges they were unaware of before receiving their hair unit. Surprises can be costly and aggravating.

Maintenance costs run about eighty dollars monthly. Also expect several charges for dyeing and adding hair to the units. These run sixty to one hundred and fifty dollars per occasion and you can expect to incur them three to four times yearly. So total maintenance costs can run about twelve hundred dollars yearly (without tips).

One of my patients sought a way to short-circuit these costs. He went to a beauty supply wholesaler after printing up cards for himself as president of a hair replacement salon. Initially he bought all the products necessary for proper maintenance such as the adhesive, the adhesive remover, the powder dye, and the shampoos used to clean the existing system. At first he was worried that he would ruin his piece, but, as we all become our own best hairdressers in order to creatively comb thinning hair, he soon became very adept at using the supplies. He also was able to remove the system on weekends for a day to "let his scalp breathe" (he wore a hat) and kept both hairpieces in proper repair and secured them well when on his scalp. This reduced his yearly maintenance costs to about three hundred dollars because he still needed to have hair added. He also claimed it increased the life of the hairpiece by a good six months.

But this was not all he did. Using his business cards he went back to the supplier to have him duplicate the hairpiece for a "client." He told the supplier that he wished to try him out for use with future clients. The replacement hair system, which certainly looked as good as the original and lasted equally as long, would have cost him three hundred dollars. He had two made up however, so he receive a discounted price of $450 for both.

With this success, he started his own business endeavor. He did this by first soliciting friends and then going to waiting rooms of salons and distributing his cards. Soon business boomed, and this hair system recipient not only had no costs for himself, but was making good money charging fair prices and delivering good service. He produced a video for his clients which explained his self hair system care.

Just today, I had a consultation with a patient who had worn hair systems for over two years. He had finally taken it off because he went to play golf on a big company social outing on a Caribbean island. He had recently had his hairpiece serviced and colored. By the time he was at the sixteenth hole everyone was looking at him peculiarly. When he looked in the mirror in the locker room he almost died from embarrassment. His hair had turned orange. So finally after over two years and nine thousand dollars of expense (according to his calculations), he was still bald and very embarrassed. He was offered a micrograft transplant for his hairline with a hairpiece behind it for another five thousand dollars, but he said no one would guarantee him that his hairpiece would not oxidize (change color) again leaving him with a two-tone head of hair. His costs would have similarly climbed substantially.

So hair systems and their maintenance can run thousands of dollars in the first year, and one to two thousand dollars in subsequent years depending on your input and ingenuity. But one fact is certain, shop around and negotiate. You can only be the winner. Most important, get a written guarantee of your costs over the next two years. If you push for it, you most likely will get the price committal, but this will only be available to you before you commit financially to a hair system purchase.

I have recently seen advertisements in New York, that

claim that for a single monthly cost, you will receive an all-inclusive package with one new hair system per year plus all maintenance costs. If you go this route, be sure of the quality of the hairpiece you will be provided with and have some escape clause written in for you if you decide to change your mind about continuing. Also beware of hidden costs such as processing or handling fees or inflated materials costs. I always love the special ads on T.V. or mail order where they beat the price you would pay locally, but the shipping and handling is so elevated that your final price for a small ticket item such as shampoo can become twice the advertised price.

Finally, beware of contractual discontinuing penalties. Read the fine print. Make sure you don't get hurt if the hair system is no longer right for you!

WHAT SHOULD A HAIR TRANSPLANT COST ME?

Now this is the jackpot question. Recently I worked with Gary Belsky from *Money* magazine on a story about the "industry" of hair loss and its replacement. Several people went "undercover" for consultations with a variety of physicians and/or clinics to determine costs for various services. What was seen was a range in price from several thousand dollars to upwards of fifty thousand dollars for hair transplant surgery. There is one clinic that clearly states in its brochure that "Remember—you get what you pay for." But do you? Elton John had a hair transplant several years ago in Europe which did not turn out very well. He spent a lot of money. He now wears a hairpiece. It is not unusual in today's climate for a consumer to become very confused.

The Apple vs. Orange Syndrome

Consider this situation. The potential patient sees advertisements for upwards of two to three thousand transplanted grafts in a single session. He or she is also led to believe that the greater the number of "grafts" transplanted, the lower the cost per graft. You now feel the more the merrier, believing that you are saving a bundle. So now you, the patient, have an economical three-thousand-graft transplant for only four dollars per graft. You have now payed the money-saving price of only twelve thousand dollars. But what have you received?

In general, when having a three-thousand-graft mega-session, each graft is a single hair. We also know that in these giant sessions, an average of only seventy percent of the grafts will take because of the length of time to perform the procedure, the delicateness of the single hair grafts, and the fatigue factor in the staff performing the tedious preparation of the grafts.

We also know that massive sessions assault the circulation of the scalp and can similarly inhibit graft take.

So now you have payed twelve thousand "economical" dollars for about twenty-one hundred hairs (out of one hundred thousand total) to be transferred to the top of your bald or balding scalp (it better be real bald if someone is going to transplant that many grafts).

Now let's compare this to the old plugs. In the old days, plugs of about four millimeters in diameter used to contain fifteen to twenty hairs each. An average session of one hundred plugs was performed on the first transplant session, normally to the frontal third of the scalp. This was only the starting session and would require subsequent sittings just to fill in the same transplanted region. This session would successfully transplant (over 95 percent take usually) about eighteen hundred hairs. At even twenty dollars per plug, the session would cost two thousand dollars. Three sessions transplanting five to six thousand hairs would cost six thousand dollars. So we've transplanted a lot more hair at a lot less cost in the old system (helping explain the lack of thickness in today's micrograft megasessions). When single hairs are spread out the result has to be thin.

This is where the apples vs. the oranges syndrome comes in. Ask not how many grafts are being transplanted in a session; instead ask how many hairs should successfully grow. Four dollars per hair (even if the success was one hundred percent) becomes very expensive compared to six hair minigrafts that generally cost about ten dollars.

Also remember, don't be naive. If you're looking for some thickness as part of your transplant result, twenty-one hundred or even three thousand hairs in Type V or VI hair loss is just not going to do it. Expect several more sessions which will substantially raise your final costs. ***Don't compare apples to oranges!***

The smart patient today will look to pay a price per session, not per graft. By this I mean the following. You have, for example, frontal hair loss. What you need to know is how many sessions it will take to achieve what you and the physician project is possible and what is the cost for each session. Also,

- Will the cost decrease in subsequent sessions especially if they become smaller in scope and are instead more like touch-up procedures?
- Can the price of the sessions change in subsequent

months because of a "price rise" or are they guaranteed?

- How many hairs (not grafts) does the physician expect to transplant each session?
- Does the price include single-hair grafts to refine the hairline or is this a separate session and cost?
- What is, if any, the cost of followups?
- Do you charge for suture removal?
- Is there an operating room fee?
- Is there an anesthesia fee?
- What if there is a problem, is care covered?
- Do followup visits for care or reevaluation cost anything?
- If you are traveling long distances (out of town) to have the procedure performed, are these any price concessions to help defer traveling and hotel costs?
- If some grafts do not take, will you replace them at no charge?
- Is there a twenty-four-hour phone reach in case of problems or do I have to seek attention at off hours at my own expense? (Do not use a physician who does not have a twenty-four-hour on-call number.)

I talked to a patient who had prior transplants. He told me that he tripped on a Sunday evening in a restaurant and caught his recent transplant on a fire extinguisher hook. He started bleeding but it stopped with pressure. He lost several grafts and the restaurant put them in a towel soaked in iced salt water for him. He called his doctor's number and got an answering machine with no option but to leave a message. He received a return phone call the next day long after he had visited a hospital emergency room. The doctors in the emergency room had no hair transplant experience and thus the grafts that had come out were discarded. It cost the patient $175 dollars for the emergency room visit and it cost the doctor a patient.

All of the above are what we call mitigating circumstances of cost. In other words it is similar to buying a car stripped and then learning just how much more it will cost with necessary equipment.

The doctor or clinic you visit can also influence the price you pay. Some have elaborate sales networks and offices which will immediately jack up the price. Others have these plus elaborate advertising in flight or other national magazines which will increase the price substantially as well. So what you decide should be predicated on result, not cost.

Another thing to beware of is the bait and switch operation. Here, you have the clinic or doctor's salesman give you a price only to discover later that this refers only to their primary physicians. If you want "top shelf," you will have to fork over two to three times the fee. This might make sense in a reasonable setting, but when the prices are crazy to start with, the final prices may truly be *out of line*. I see this constantly in the setting of physician confidence. Patients are told, "You must use me" in order to obtain the best result. The price, though, as it is relayed, is of little consequence to your result. Unfortunately, the result may be disproportionate to the price.

Another caveat is the nonrefundable deposit. Here you are asked to pay a portion if not all of the fee for your upcoming procedure upfront. Now this can be a routine and acceptable practice because the physician is reserving his time and facility for your procedure. He has expenses and must cover them. Where it is not acceptable is when you discover that a portion if not all of the fee is nonrefundable, even if you cancel well in advance. You may instead be issued a credit towards a future procedure you do not want.

Beware of contracts—my patients pay for their procedure the day I perform it. I do not ask for deposits unless the patient has repeatedly cancelled his appointment at the last minute. I consult with my patients personally so I do not have a salesman's salary or commission structure to deal with.

So aside from these caveats, your hair transplant should, in reasonable hands, cost from two to four thousand dollars per session for the initial one or two large sessions. Smaller subsequent sessions should cost less. Your total cost should not exceed ten to twelve thousand dollars unless you are very bald (and still a candidate) or you wish subsequent additional transplanting such as achieving as much densification of results as is feasible. In the old days we called these people "plug junkies." There was no stopping their desire to add more and more hair in even the most obscure spots. I remember one patient who drove me crazy by returning every six to eight weeks with several spots he marked by himself on his scalp for me to fill. His wife would beg me to discourage him as his result looked fine, but the more I discouraged him, the more he wanted additional work. I finally flatly refused to do more and his wife served him with divorce papers. He stopped the transplanting but still calls to ask when he can resume.

Other than the transplant price, your maintenance is a haircut. This is one of the beauties of growing back your own hair. Other costs only come into play if additional hair is lost in the future. It costs nothing in my office to stop by and say hello.

WHAT SHOULD A SCALP REDUCTION COST?

Scalp reductions vary in design, complexity, and thus price. I have had patients come in with prior reductions that they paid five thousand dollars for and I have seen patients who only paid one thousand dollars. In either case, the patients didn't necessarily get what they paid for.

Another caveat is the multiple reduction recommendation. Here, although the price for each procedure may sound reasonable, the plan is to perform three or more scalp reductions. In general, I have seen patients who looked good after their first reduction, fair after their second one, and worse than before they began after the third. They paid two thousand to twenty-five hundred dollars for each procedure and it will now cost them thousands more to undo the result.

I have one patient who came to me after having a large midline reduction where he had a balloon inserted during the procedure to stretch the scalp. He sat at the surgeon's office for six hours with this balloon inserted, waiting for the final reduction surgery. During this time, he had an intravenous delivering fluids to him and was monitored by a nurse anesthetist. The result was not very impressive after reviewing his pre-op pictures and he had definite evidence of stretchback. This in itself was not as big a problem as his bill, which amounted to *eight thousand dollars*. The breakdown was as follows.

Blood tests pre-op	$350.00
Preprocedure exam	$250.00
O.R. fee	$500.00
Equipment fee (I.V., balloon, etc.)	$500.00

Nurse anesthetist	$1500.00
Surgery	$4500.00
Recovery room	$400.00
Total	$8000.00

He told me that he was never quoted other fees than that for the surgery alone and he was thus very agitated with the final tab. Add to that the poor result and I was obviously talking to a very unhappy patient who was now significantly poorer.

So before I tell you what you should pay, let me tell you what financial questions I think you should ask before scheduling the surgery—in other words, what you should be aware of.

- What is the surgical fee?
- What other extra costs are there?
- Do I require anesthesia?
- If I do or may, is there a fee and how much?
- What equipment must I pay for?
- What happens if there is a complication?
- What if it doesn't work, do I pay again?
- Is there followup cost?
- Do you charge for suture removal?
- When must I cancel by?
- Is there a cancellation fee?

When you are finished, ask not only for a breakdown of each amount, but also for a written summary of the costs. By now it goes without saying that you should talk this over with the physician, but also remember that you *can negotiate* the price. I have never charged an O.R. fee when procedures are performed in my office. This is what I call my rent. This is *my* overhead, not yours, and should figure in to the price of procedure. If a person wanted intravenous or general anesthesia as has rarely happened (and is not needed) I will let them make their own arrangements with my recommended nurse anesthetist or surgery center. No surgeon should charge for followup or suture removal on his own surgical procedure. This is deemed in most states to be unethical. I constantly am seeing patients nickel-and-dimed with these extras and quite honestly, it is a blight on the profession.

Thus, scalp reductions (without expanders or extenders) should cost you between fifteen hundred and two thousand dollars depending on the size of the procedure. It should be handled in one or two surgeries; beware of three or more unless yours is a special case. Your followup should be free and if a revision of the result is necessary because of a complication such as stretchback, this should not result in an additional cost to you.

In my practice, all of our scalp reductions are performed with a special anchoring suture that helps prevent stretchback, Clinical studies confirm the effectiveness of this method. The special PDS suture material costs me about seven dollars. I do not endeavor to pass this cost on to the patient.

Reductions fees in my office are seventeen hundred and fifty dollars. There are no extra costs (I pay my own rent and staff costs). Complications, although rare, are handled by us at no cost to the patient. Repeat scalp reductions are only performed in very bald patients and my fee for the second reduction will decrease to fifteen hundred dollars. I do not charge for suture removal, and I provide the necessary medicines (except Tylenol #3 if necessary) free to the patients as well as any gauze or topical medications that may be required. Besides the cost, I don't feel that people want to go from a procedure to a pharmacy, they would rather just go home.

Scalp reductions which include extenders or expanders are a horse of a different color.

Here the patient is required to pay for the price of the device (usually five hundred to one thousand dollars) as well as at least two surgical procedures one to two months apart. Patients tell me that the cost of the procedures run approximately two to three thousand dollars each and repeat reductions (with the extra costs of equipment) are often the rule. This can bring your total cost for scalp reduction with expansion or extension up to ten to fifteen thousand dollars. Now it's time to add the cost of hair transplantation to this.

I can't repeat often enough how you should ask for an itemized list of costs. If you need two separate procedures, remember this is four surgeries (one to put in expander or extender and a second to remove the device and complete the scalp reduction four to eight weeks later. Complications, sometimes including hospitalization, may cost you extra especially if your health insurance (as is the case in many patients) is poor or nonexistent.

So if this is the route you wish to take, make sure you are financially ready to handle the journey. This is not the type of surgery that can be stopped midstream and forgotten about. And remember to add the costs of hair transplantation to the final cost because this will be a necessary completion to the procedure. This is why so many of us now perform the curvilinear scalp reduction. It not only reduces the immediate cost of the procedure, but also helps limit the cost of any necessary subsequent hair restoration work.

Also, be aware that scalp reductions performed in the midline including those with extenders will require a slot correction procedure. If you do not prenegotiate this in your procedural price, it is conceivable for you to add several thousand dollars to the cost of your procedure. If the slot correction does not work the first time, additional procedures may be required costing thousands more.

WHAT WILL A SCALP LIFT COST?

Scalp lifting, as I have explained earlier, is a radical form of scalp reduction. In today's terms, it also requires more than one surgical procedure because it is necessary to first tie off the occipital arteries several weeks prior to the scalp lifting surgery. The actual surgery itself requires intravenous anesthesia and this should be given only by an experienced nurse anesthetist or anesthesiologist. It certainly can and should be performed in an office with proper facilities including recovery rooms. The anesthesia will probably be extra, but the room and followup should not.

Patients post–scalp lifting have reported to me that their cost breakdowns are generally five hundred dollars for the precare including ligation of the arteries, and up to ten thousand dollars for the surgery plus anesthesia. Postoperative care is generally included, but complications are not. Repeat procedures are generally not needed, but subsequent transplantation of hair always is.

Revisions of any necrosed (poorly taken) area are generally included depending on the surgeon. Remember, revision or correction of severe complications may not only be costly, it may not be possible. Always make sure that the surgeon you choose to perform this procedure is well experienced in its execution. This is not the procedure you want some newly experienced doctor to perform on you.

Total cost of scalp lifting plus hair transplantation will be in the neighborhood of twenty to thirty thousand dollars.

WHAT SHOULD SCALP FLAPS COST?

It is not uncommon for me to see patients who have spent forty to fifty thousand dollars in surgical costs plus another twenty thousand dollars in transportation and housing costs. This is before the patient even finishes with hair transplantation. Postoperative costs, unless the patient remains in the locale of the surgeon, will generally be extra. Often, the patient is forced to fly back to the location (many of these are in California) to have postoperative care rendered. This is because many local doctors will not wish to render the postoperative care because of lack of familiarity with the procedure. Complications can be more common than more conventional procedures and often require the patient to return to the rendering surgeon. Loss of income is also a problem for many as patients are often forced to take a leave of absence from their work because of their interim appearance. Anesthesia adds another cost, and general anesthesia is definitely required.

So if the flap route is the one you wish to take, expect the potential costs of completing the job to be possibly six figures. If you can't afford this, don't even consider it. If you can afford this, be sure it's the way you wish to go.

Once again, as mentioned before, be careful of cancellation fees or other financial obligations. Have your costs itemized and be sure any additional possibilities are similarly outlined. Get the name of doctors in your home locale who will render your aftercare and call them beforehand for cost breakdown as well as their experience with prior patients having similar procedures.

This is major surgery, so do not take it lightly.

WHAT ARE THE COSTS OF SOME OTHER PROCEDURES?

Other procedures, to me, are a grouping of some unusual methods of hair replacement. For example, there is a recent system of implanting metal clips in the scalp to help attach a hairpiece. In this case, the surgical cost can be two to three thousand dollars not including the cost of the hairpiece. Remember, this is a way to attach a hairpiece, not a surgical cure for baldness.

In Japan, it is still legal to perform surgical hair implantation. Here artificial fibers are sewn into people's scalps to simulate real hair. In the past, the fibers could not be readily removed causing profound difficulties. This led to them being outlawed in this country. The new implant fiber techniques, although having their own complication rate, allow the fibers to be easily removed.

Other physicians familiar with this procedure report the costs to be in the fifteen- to thirty-thousand-dollar range. This does not include ongoing medical attention plus the maintenance and replacement costs of the implanted fibers (they have to be replaced every three to six months). I would not recommend this procedure for man or beast.

A cure developed recently hovers at the edge of legality in the U.S. It involves implanting human hairs rather than the outlawed artificial fibers. When problems occurred, the parties responsible for the procedure shifted to having metal cylinders with human hair inserted throughout the bald area. This resulted in a head of intermittent human hairs implanted through the scalp. One patient that I had seen actually set off the metal detector in the airport in France while returning to the U.S. after the surgery. The cost of this procedure varies from forty to one hundred thousand dollars and this does not include ongoing maintenance. You also must pay traveling costs and costs of medical attention for the complications. This is a radical and I believe a somewhat dangerous approach to treating hair loss. At best, it is ridiculously expensive.

ELEVEN

WHAT IF MY HAIR LOSS IS NOT ON MY SCALP?

Alopecia doesn't only occur on the scalp, and hair loss elsewhere can also affect our appearance and our lifestyles.

I once had a patient who came to see me about a hair transplant. I looked at him and thought that either he had the best most undetectable hairpiece I had ever seen, or his visit to me was premature. After questioning him for a few minutes I soon discovered my focus was predicated on my belief that all those who see me come for scalp hair loss. Well in this case I was talking to an Israeli rabbinical student who had traveled from the Middle East for help. It seemed that he had suffered a bout with alopecia areata (spotty hair loss of unknown cause) several years before, and although most of the hair regrew, he suffered permanent loss on the right side of his face where his beard should be. This might not be a problem for a smooth shaver, but it is, however, one for an orthodox rabbi. He was told that without a thick beard, his future could not be assured. I referred the problem to Dr. Alan Engler, a plastic surgeon with extensive facial experience, and together we successfully transplanted hair to his right beard region. I have performed many of these procedures since then, and found that the latest technology has made the procedure and the result more natural and more predictable.

About six years ago, I was fortunate enough to hire a medical assistant from Taiwan. In addition to bringing a great deal of expertise and a desire to work hard to the practice, she sought to educate me about the vast numbers of Asians who lacked both eyebrow and eyelash hair. She showed (and translated) advertisements in many of the Chinese language newspapers targeting those women self-conscious about thinning eyebrows and lashes. Most of these advertisements pointed to tattooing as a means of treatment, but one or two talked about the use of hair transplantation. Indeed, the original hair replacement surgery was developed for just this purpose.

The premise for much of the subsequent work in hair replacement surgery centered on the prevalence of patchy eyebrow growth in numerous Asian women. Although much of the early correction involved modified standard punch graft transplanting, the latest techniques have offered the best results.

WHAT CAUSES THINNING EYEBROWS?

One's genes are the usual but not the only cause of thinning eyebrows. When I was a medical student and assigned to the emergency room, I was always warned about treating cuts in the eyebrow region. It seems that if you shave the hair on eyebrows even in order to suture a cut, the hair may not grow back.

Other causes of permanent hair loss in the eyebrow region involve aggressive eyebrow hair tweezing, burns, trauma, alopecia areata (which can occur anywhere), and even leprosy. The cosmetic effect especially on young women can be devastating. Certain forms of tattooing for enhancement of eyebrows have also been known to cause permanent hair loss, but this practice still continues.

HOW CAN I REPAIR THINNING EYEBROWS?

Although plug hair transplantation can certainly help, it still has many of the limitations in the eyebrow region that it has when performed on the frontal hairline. Plugs were never good at creating a transition zone for the hairline and instead would often cause a desert to forest effect, which draws attention to an unnatural hairline. The difference for scalp hair is that it can be combed in various ways to help conceal the hairline. This is not true in the eyebrow region. Here there is a direct view of the hair-bearing area and its borders similar to a bird's eye view of scalp hair. Thus plugs in the eyebrow region can indeed by very unforgiving.

Another important factor which becomes paramount to success in eyebrow hair restoration is the hair growth angle. Eyebrow hair grows at less than a fifteen-degree angle above the skin, almost parallel with it. In addition, it is vital to realize that in each eyebrow, hair direction will vary with the portion of the eyebrow. Think of the center of the eyebrow as a straight line. Hair above it grows slightly upward and hair below it grows in a slightly downward direction. The most central portion of the eyebrow grows upward only.

To reconstruct this correctly, plugs are almost entirely useless. In addition, plugs may cause cobblestoning (bumps), which will make the result unsightly and give the patient more problems than they came to the doctor with.

Dr. Choi's single hair inserter is nice for this because it "injects" living single hairs into the eyebrow region in the direction the surgeon desires. It also, unlike plugs, does not first remove a bald area of skin, therefore it does not create a defect. The hairs can be injected close together by the experienced surgeon. I have performed several of these procedures quite successfully. Most recently, I had a famous Chinese rock star (from Taiwan) who came to repair her eyebrows. She had had a part in a major motion picture where she played a future alien who had no eyebrows. Instead of having them waxed, plucked, or shaven closely, she had electrolysis performed on her eyebrow region. The result was very successful for her alien outer space role, but was far less profitable for her return to human civilization. She was now forced to stencil in eyebrows and even tried wearing two eyebrow "hairpieces" to hide the problem. She came to me for help.

I was successful in transplanting several hundred single hairs back into the eyebrow region. Interestingly, most grew immediately unlike what usually occurs with scalp hair transplant. The only drawback is that she must cut the hair periodically as it will continue to grow to the same length the hair would have in its original location.

This helps point out the necessity of choosing donor hair very carefully in eyebrow surgery. What I do now is use high neck hair or hair from just behind the ear region because it is here where the hair most closely simulates the hair color and texture of eyebrows. Thicker higher hair may look peculiar in a facial location.

More recently a new knife blade and handle have been developed by Dr. Jim Arnold in California that facilitates eyebrow transplantation. With this device, we can set the blade length to perfectly match the length of the hair and root we are to transplant. Think of the blade as a pointy fat needle which not only pushes the skin apart where the hair is to be inserted, but also dilates (stretches) the skin, making insertion easier. Angle here is easier to achieve. The hairs can also be placed closer together than with the Choi inserter. Results have been excellent.

ARE THERE COMPLICATIONS?

Any surgery can have complications, but there have been relatively few here. The main problem is generally a direct result of an inexperienced surgeon who should not be performing the procedure.

Recently, a new advertisement popped up where the surgeon (who had only an internship and no formal residency) claimed that his results were "better than natural." He also touted his ability to reconstruct eyebrows, eyelashes, and other facial hair defects. His lack of formal training makes one nervous enough, but the patient who came to me after having his procedure scared me even more. Hair direction in the eyebrow region was ignored. Hair grew, but this young women looked like Groucho Marx. She was depressed and desperate. The hair was dark and unruly.

What I did here was first to send for her electrolysis. There was no way to correct the problem without first removing the culprit. Hair selection was poor and these coarse dark hairs were unforgiving. Similarly there was no way to correct the improper hair direction. So in my opinion it was best to start with a clean slate.

Electrolysis was staged over a four-month period and then she was given another two months to heal. Most of the hairs were removed, and she wore a medicated makeup (colored) to hide the defect. After six months we were ready for the repair. I chose donor hair from behind her ears and first performed a test session in the corners of both eyebrows. Because of the prior surgery, I was worried about scarring and growth. The hair grew immediately and well, so we were ready to proceed.

After several sessions (I worked slowly because of all the prior work) I was able to achieve a good cosmetic effect. She was happy and her life, which was put on hold for almost a year, proceeded again.

Again, you must check the experience of the surgeon who will be performing the procedure. You must see his results and most importantly talk to him, *not a sales representative*. Remember, only you will wear the results.

Other complications such as infection probably exist, but I have never seen or heard of it in eyebrow surgery. Preventative antibiotics and antiseptic aftercare should alway be included postoperatively.

Poor growth is more a function of poor technique. This was especially true with the old plug method where poorly angled plugs transplanted the hairs without the roots, thus causing no growth. Similarly, poor growth can also be attributed to poor preparation of the single hairs to be transplanted. Overmanipulation of these delicate hairs can certainly damage them and thereby significantly decrease the number that take.

Cobblestoning was a function of plug use because the donor hairs in the plugs had roots deeper than those in the more shallow eyebrow region. As a result, the plug would be too deep and cause surface elevation. It can be corrected easily, however, with electric needle dessication (shaving) of the elevated surface skin.

Loss of sensation will generally occur locally but will

usually recover fully over a several week period. This is very true with the single hair insertions as no surface nerves are cut as they could be with plugs. This is, therefore, not a problem.

Swelling is temporary and is the result of any surgical procedure or injury to a region.

CAN EYELASH TRANSPLANTATION BE DONE?

As I have mentioned earlier in this book, the original ideas for modern hair transplantation originated in the Far East. They came about not just for eyebrows and scalp hair, but to help solve the problem of poor eyelash development seen in Oriental women as well. As is appropriate, the doctors with the most experience in this field developed it in Asia (Korea).

Doctors Choi and Kim report success using Dr. Choi's special hair inserter. They utilize donor hair from the nape of the neck where it is finer and does not grow at the rate of healthy scalp hair. They then take special precautions to protect the eye from any potential injury. After this they insert the new hairs one by one into the eyelid itself. Care must be taken to preserve direction of the hairs as you don't want the hairs in the upper lid growing down over your field of vision any more than you want the lower hairs growing upward. The hairs must be trimmed from time to time because otherwise they will grow longer than normal eyelashes (they still think they are in the nape of the neck).

I must admit I have no personal experience with eyelash transplantation. I must also further admit that I don't want any either. The idea of it frightens me. This is an area I would caution anyone to enter very slowly. I would insist an ophthalmologist be present to protect my eyeballs and socket and would demand to see several patients and talk to them before proceeding. I would only use a physician who performs these routinely. As I have said earlier, I recently saw an advertisement touting the skills of a physician to perform every chapter of hair transplantation including eyelashes. I know his experience as well as his training is limited and I would be frightened for anyone using him for eyelash transplants.

ARE THERE COMPLICATIONS?

In all of my research, I could not find anyone discussing complications from this procedure, but there have to be. My personal communications with other physicians in the field have revealed cyst formation on the eyelids requiring hair removal as well localized infections requiring antibiotics and sometimes hair removal. This is not a procedure I would take lightly.

WHAT OTHER AREAS CAN BE TRANSPLANTED?

When I was a surgical resident at Columbia Presbyterian Medical Center in New York in the 70's, we were a referral center for many developmental problems that could not be handled elsewhere. One of these was a situation where a baby was born with its bladder outside its body, a condition known as exstrophy of the bladder. Surgery was required to repair this within the first twenty-four to forty-eight hours of life or else the bladder would "dry out" and have to be permanently removed. I was on the repair team. In order to repair this condition, flaps of skin had to be rotated from the baby's sides (flanks) to cover the defect in the pubic area made by reinserting the bladder in its proper position. This worked fine, functionally, but cosmetic problems would begin at puberty. Here, the normal pubic hair would grow in a V pattern because other skin had been brought in to fill in the center of the pubic region. So now you have an adolescent with abnormally shaped pubic hair. These young adults suffered from this psychologically and required counseling.

In 1978 I was asked if hair transplantation might work in these cases. I was uncertain because the prior surgery had probably left much scar tissue and although I knew the transplanted skin would take, I didn't know if the hair follicles would. Nonetheless, I wanted to help so I decided to try.

My first attempt was on a fourteen-year-old girl who had refused to shower in locker rooms or even date because of the problem. She was shy to the point of not wanting me to even see the area. She had the classic V-shaped pubic hair growth pattern and it was my job to close in the V. We performed her procedure in the operating room taking special precautions to avoid infection in the scarred pubic region (the scalp on the other hand, rarely becomes infected). I transplanted thirty medium-size plugs of hair from her donor sites and placed them into receptor sites much smaller in diameter. I did this to squeeze the hairs closer together and cause the hairs to grow frizzy. She did fine postoperatively, but we still had to wait three to four months to see the results.

Well it worked, and I went on to transplanting additional plugs in the region to recreate the pubic hair's natural growth pattern. The only long-term complication was the need to trim the hair as it grew longer. This procedure became finally routine in these children and I must say it helped cure a horrible psychological handicap.

Another aspect of pubic hair transplantation involves women with just plain thin hair in the region. In Roman times as well as presently, women would wear pubic hair wigs known as Merkens. They would glue them on to enhance the appearance of the region. I have had several women asking for pubic hair transplantation for thinning hair in the region, and after proper screening for donor hair as well as discussion of expectation, I have performed several. This is a good procedure. Although I doubted you would ever see an advertisement for this, with the latest ads for penile enlargement flooding the newsprint, nothing seems off limits. Perhaps the field of genito-urinary hair transplantion will soon be a new specialty.

CAN I HAVE MY CHEST MADE HAIRY?

This fortunately is not a request that I see very often. Although I have never attempted to do this, I have talked to colleagues who have. In the past, plugs transplanted to the chest area could cause bumpiness as well as sporadic growth. Numbness over parts of the chest from cutting surface nerves also occurred regularly.

Today, single-hair transplantation works much better with far fewer problems. The hairs are inserted singly and space is left between individual hairs. Growth appears excellent and few if any complications result. There is no bumpiness and the hairs grow in sooner than twelve weeks in most cases. As mentioned before, the only drawback is that the hairs will need to be trimmed as they grow longer, but this is not a big problem.

I must say that although many men have asked me to transplant hair from their "virile" chest, none have ever asked me to reverse the role. To answer the question you are probably thinking, the chest is a lousy donor site for hair transplantation. The hairs are far apart and do not look like scalp hair.

In summary, let me say that the most recent developments in my field have allowed us to transfer living growing hair to areas we never thought possible and to get results that are simply terrific. When you match the right experienced surgeon with the right procedure, you will usually get the right result with limited but fixable complications. Always keep this principle in mind.

TWELVE

WHAT DOES THE FUTURE HOLD FOR HAIR REPLACEMENT?

Hair replacement in the twenty-first century may well become the largest focus amongst today's cosmetically oriented population. This is predicated on the fact that hair transplantation is now the most commonly performed cosmetic procedure according to the American Academy of Cosmetic Surgery. In order to attempt to answer this very difficult question for you, I will need to break it down into the categories covered in the chapters throughout this book. Although I don't have a crystal ball, I've polled the experts in each field to try to bring you their predictions.

WHAT IS THE FUTURE OF OVER-THE-COUNTER CREAMS AND LOTIONS?

The easiest way to answer this question is to look at the past. Creams, lotions, ointments, miracle cures, and the hucksters who promote them will be around far longer than you or I. Just like my young twins being fascinated with the magic of Cinderella or Aladdin, our hope for a magical cure will always have many of us "give it a try."

Recently, I was approached by some people who asked me to help promote a new "special shampoo" tested in Europe with great success. It apparently unclogs not just the pores, but also degunks the swollen hair bulb. Unsubstantiated clinical trials have shown 70 to 80 percent effectiveness in restoring hair growth. Sounds good—probably some of you are waiting for me to give you the name of the product so you can run out and try it. Well don't bother. I reviewed the "research" and found that they tested it on people with nonhereditary hair loss. They found the same regrowth of hair they would have seen if any other product or none at all was used.

This product, which will be released in the next year, will probably generate a lot of money but not a lot of results. It is nothing but another Cinderella story, minus the happy ending.

Save your money—there are many more effective remedies on the horizon.

WHAT IS THE FUTURE OF MEDICAL HAIR REPLACEMENT?

Since the financial success of minoxidil for the Upjohn Co., many other drug companies have now entered the race to produce a successful treatment for hair loss. It is important to realize that most of these therapies have two goals: preventing hair loss and restoring hair follicles not yet dead. The idea of reviving dead follicles is about as practical as throwing a miracle cream on a grave and expecting someone to wake up.

So to look at the twenty-first century, I will try to overview some of the categories of experimental drugs now being tested for debut after the start of the next millennium.

Five Alpha Reductase Inhibitors

These drugs are to prevent testosterone from being converted into 5DHT, the culprit in hereditary hair loss. The pill version (proscar) which I mentioned in an earlier chapter, is being tested currently, but several side-effects have been noticed. The next generation of this drug would logically be a topical version which could be absorbed to the level of your hair's living root and provide protection for it.

Studies have been conducted in macaque monkeys (who suffer hereditary hair loss) over a two-and-a-quarter-year period. A topical form of the 5 alpha reductase inhibitor was applied to a group of balding monkeys and this was compared to another group who were not treated. The topical blocker was deemed effective in slowing or stopping the progression of hair loss. Another study then went on to compare the use of Proscar alone to Proscar combined with topical minoxidil. Here, too, it was deemed the combination was considered more effective than either drug used alone.

So this is one of the categories of drugs we will see after the year 2000. Testing is of course preliminary and side-effects are unknown. Further clinical trials are certainly needed before the Food and Drug Administration allows testing on humans to begin. These last for three to five years, so don't expect to run to the pharmacy or your physician and be able to use these drugs anytime soon. Remember, the FDA is there to protect us sometimes against ourselves.

Androgen (Testosterone) Blockers

This therapy is given in pill form in an effort to block male hormone levels. This is really a regimen for female pattern hair loss for it is not really practical to block testosterone in males. Studies using these drugs are being complicated by only the need to monitor blood iron levels as well as levels of Vitamin B_{12}. Although hair counts in the very first trials showed increases in women with female pattern hair loss, the side-effects are not known and long-term therapy may prove dangerous. After a long sorting out and testing procedure, these drugs may come to market in the fight to treat female pattern baldness.

DHT (Dihydrotestosterone) Inhibitors (Pill form)

DHT inhibitors are also aimed at female pattern hair loss. In this category, several drugs such as cimetidine (Tagamet) which currently is used to treat ulcer disease, have been found to block DHT competitively. Only one trial that I'm aware of has been conducted in a small series of female patients, but results were encouraging. The problem is that hair loss after Tagamet use has also been reported. The next step of course will be much larger studies with an eye towards dosage and side-effects. Look for DHT inhibitors on the shelves in a few years as another medical treatment in the drug companies' race to win their share of the mega-dollars spent on hair loss.

Topical DHT Blockers

Here the race seems to be heating up. Years ago I was one of the victims of the promises made of using a prescription medication with "a special penetrating agent" available from a physician only and touted as a topical DHT blocker for the scalp. I had to clog my shower drain and scoop up hairs daily (in order to determine if I was losing more than the average fifty to one hundred hairs per day) and neatly place them in plastic bags that were dated. The result was I spent a lot of money on a useless cream and even more money on plastic bags. At that point the only thing found effective to stop falling hair was the floor. But the idea was good and many companies have persisted in their effort to find an effective topical dihydrotestosterone blocker. This then allows males to use the medication as it is no longer delivered systemically (in the bloodstream as a pill would necessarily do).

One topical DHT blocker that has come to my attention during the writing of this book is Kevis. This combination of vasodilator (which opens blood channels) and H.U.C.P. (a biological complex containing hyaluronic acid, which is a DHT blocker) has been tried in Europe with reported but to my mind unsubstantiated success. Since all of the ingredients are FDA approved physicians in the United States can dispense the medicine. I am first, however, embarking on my own clinical test with my patients to see if this is fact or fiction. I've been in touch with several dermatologists in Italy who swear by the medicine, but they also have financial connections to the pharmaceutical company manufacturing it. For this reason I am helping to coordinate an effort amongst responsible hair replacement physicians in this country to do responsible testing with followup. This will involve hair counts and consistent photography. If it works, then perhaps the next century will bring an effective hair loss preventer to market. If not, it will join the myriad of hopefuls that have come and gone. I will do my best to keep all informed, but to date there is no convincing effect.

WHAT IS THE FUTURE OF HAIRPIECES AND SYSTEMS?

First, let me say that hairpieces will always have a place in society. There will always be that portion of our population that will either not be a candidate for or simply not want surgical hair replacement. There will also always be a category of patients who will need temporary hairpiece coverage for temporary hair loss related to drug treatment or accident. So to say that the day of the hair system has come and gone is not true.

What is true is that hair systems will have to continue to improve. New, even lighter based systems for those totally bald on top with more secure, less irritating adhesives are currently in the process of development. Hair systems are also being developed that really do allow one's own remaining hair to be integrated with the replacement hair, but are also sturdy and hold up well.

Further developments are in the works to produce synthetic hair that resists losing its body (wave or curl) after getting wet. The "hair" for systems is improving but it still has a long way to go.

The trend in the future also seems to shifting back to hair extensions. Very light clusters of hair are being secured to thinning hair to add volume and thickness. The problem has always been that the weight of the added hair combined with the weakness of the thinning hair has accelerated hair breakage and loss. The new additions being tested are much lighter and less fragile. We'll see in the future how they work.

The biggest trend for the future, however, is the combined procedure. At meetings now, it is not unusual for me to find hair replacement center people coming to talk to hair replacement surgeons. Meetings are similarly helping physicians to learn about hairpieces and systems so they can offer a combination to the patient who just doesn't have the hair or the desire to go through a completed surgical procedure.

My feeling is that although people are beginning to transplant hairlines and placing hairpieces behind them, the trend will progress more to transplanting hairlines and side parts and putting a much smaller piece on top to complete the job. This would be beneficial to those wishing it in several ways. All visible hairlines and part lines would be natural, growing hair. This would also allow the patient/client to comb his own hair into the hair system. Naturally growing hair would similarly greatly aid the ability of the wearer to camouflage the hairpiece and would also allow for a much more free lifestyle in terms of swimming and sports.

The combination procedure would also allow the patient to wear a much smaller and less expensive hairpiece which he could remove at night if he wished and reapply in the morning by himself, thereby significantly reducing maintenance time and cost.

Finally, the combined procedure would give the patient the option either to add some more hair surgically in the future, or to remove the piece and still look normal. It would simply not look great having a small front fringe and nothing behind it, but with part hair combed over, the patient would just look like he is balding.

One other aspect the future of hair pieces holds is decreased cost. When I was younger I remember seeing a watch that actually told the time digitally instead of by the traditional two hands. I was fascinated by it. The wearer told me that he had spent almost five hundred (1970's) dollars for this one-of-a kind item. The same watch today sells for less than ten dollars and is often a promotional giveaway. Similarly, for hairpieces, as supply increases along with competition, price will decrease and quality will improve. The aspect of feeling "held hostage" by the people who sold you the system will also diminish as self-help kits with adhesive dissolver, new adhesive easy to self-apply, hair system shampoo, and even simple color touch-up dyes become available. The two industries of surgical and nonsurgical hair replacement are beginning to and will continue to overlap even further in the future.

WHAT IS THE FUTURE OF HAIR TRANSPLANTATION?

Every year seems to bring newer techniques and improvements in the types of hair-bearing grafts as well as in the instruments used to transplant them. What I feel will occur in the future is a better system for harvesting the grafts and making them more precise to fit the sites. This is already happening with excellent results by those physicians using the multiblade knife with different size partitions to perfectly match the size of a graft to the size of a linear site. But one large company with its engineers are looking to the future and are also working on an instrument that will create the site, cut a perfect size graft, and even insert it correctly with the press of a button. The instrument will be disposable but will not be expensive. I'm presently involved as one of several clinical settings where it will be tested.

What's most interesting for the future of transplanting is what we are seeing written and talked about now, the swing back to the larger graft. People want hair density as well as naturalness. The new grafts combined with even the older larger ones can provide both. I've never abandoned larger grafts and it's gratifying to see so many responsible hair replacement surgeons shift back towards using them. The difference that I see coming is the more widespread use of the larger linear graft. Larger grafts do not have to look pluggy, and linear grafts (thin strips of single hairs in a line) are certainly the example of this.

Laser hair transplants will probably go the way of the dinosaur. Even now, responsible physicians who have touted and tested the system are beginning to predict its demise. You see, laser hair transplants is really a misnomer. The laser is only used to make a cut on the scalp. It in no way has any connection with the preparation or delivery of the hair-bearing grafts from the patient's donor area. Growth is unpredictable and the grafts are only of small size. Linear grafting should replace this.

The beauty of the future of hair transplantation is that transplants from the past and present are able to be upgraded (like a computer) as new technology evolves. My original transplants are over twenty years old, but with the newer linear and single hair grafts I've recently had added to my own locks, I'm able to comb my hair straight back. This allows my result to look almost as good as any I can turn out today. Newer instrumentation and inventions will probably facilitate the procedure by making it quicker and more comfortable for the patient, but I find it hard to imagine it being so much better from a result point of view.

WHAT IS THE FUTURE OF SCALP REDUCTION?

I used to perform eight to ten scalp reductions weekly. I now perform one or two per month. This is because the indications for scalp reductions are decreasing as the technology to transplant hair in the crown area is vastly improving.

Scalp reductions will be performed with less frequency because they will be reserved for those that are very bald in the crown and not for men or women with only thinning hair.

WHAT IS THE FUTURE OF FLAPS?

Since I don't believe they have a true present, it's hard for me to see their future. In fairness though, flap surgery today is light years ahead of where it was even five years ago. I think flaps can have a future only if they are used sparingly and not placed too low in the frontal region. A single flap can give excellent density but it must be combined with single hair grafting in the future to make a natural hairline if it is to survive. So I predict that flaps will be less aggressive and placed further back on the scalp in the future.

WHAT ABOUT CLONING HAIR— WILL WE SEE THIS ANY TIME SOON?

Recently an article was published by Drs. Choi and Kim about the regenerative power of a human hair. They took a healthy hair, removed its bulb (root), and grafted it onto the same patient's leg. The result was that the hair sheath was able to form its own new root. The hair bulb was always thought necessary to grow a hair back, and this was the first demonstration that it was not so.

Although limited, this very recent experiment was the first step in developing a method to copy. The next step will be to see if these results can be duplicated by other experimenters as well. It will also be necessary to see if the duplication process can work in vitro (outside of the body in, for example, a petrie dish) or if it must occur in vivo (on the patient himself). Techniques for duplicating large quantities of hair must next be developed, assuring that the process even works. Prior attempts at cloning have not been very consistent at replicating a healthy hair. What this means for us is that in our lifetime we will probably not see human hair cloned successfully, even if the early experiments work. Fortunately, the future's alternatives look very bright.

EPILOGUE

Many years ago I was told that if I wanted to save my hair (I was rapidly losing it), I should get a shoebox. Well we've come a long way since then in both saving and replacing it.

Although research in treatments of hair loss are going on even as you read this chapter, one thought must be kept in mind: There is no miracle cure that will be here tomorrow—so don't be fooled. Most treatments on the horizon may help (such as Rogaine) but they will not be the instant result that we all desire.

Remember, medications may have side-effects, so it may pay to wait for a bit before trying every new fad, medication, "cure," or treatment out there.

The Food and Drug Administration, slow as it may be, is there to protect the public from dangerous side-effects as well as to make a company prove that a treatment really can work.

Let me end by mentioning an article brought in by a patient with thin donor hair. The article is entitled, "New hope for baldies—HAIR transplants from corpses."

He asked me if it was really true and has sought second opinions on its veracity. People want a miracle—*there are none!*

GLOSSARY OF HAIR TRANSPLANT TERMS

Circular graft: (plug) the old standard round graft of any size inserted into a smaller receptor site.

Donor area: the area from which the transplant hair is taken. (This is usually the back or sides of the scalp.)

Harvesting: removing the donor hair strips.

Laser slit: a cut made by a fast-pulsed CO_2 laser that vaporizes a thin area of tissue, thereby creating a slot site for a transplant graft.

Linear graft: a graft of single-hair diameter whose length varies with the numbers of hairs desired for transplanting (the larger the graft, the more the numbers of hairs). The hairs are in a line and not a clump like the old circular plugs.

Maxigraft: more than six hairs per graft.

Micrograft: one to three hairs per graft.

Minigraft: four to six hairs per graft.

Recipient area: the bald area receiving the transplanted hair.

Single hair graft: a single hair transplanted to a bald area.

Slit grafting: a cut into which a hair transplant graft is inserted from which no bald or balding tissue is removed.

BIBLIOGRAPHY

BOOKS

Growing New Hair! Margo (Autumn Press, Brookline Massachusetts, 1980).

Hair Techniques and Alternatives to Baldness. John Mayhew (Trado-Medic Books, New York, 1983).

Consumer Reports Press, Neil Sadick, M.D. ''Your Hair: How to Keep It'' (1993).

Hair Replacement, Surgical, and Medical. Dow B. Stough M.D. and Robert Haber M.D. (Mosby-Year Books, Inc., St. Louis, 1996).

Stedmans Medical Dictionary. (Twenty-first Edition, Williams and Wilkins Co., Baltimore, 1966).

Clinics in Dermatology, ''Androgenetic Alopecia: From Empiricism to Knowledge'' (Elsevier Science Publishing, Oct.–Dec. 1988, Vol.6, No.4).

PERIODICALS

Dermatologic Surgery. Monthly publication of Research Articles, Elsevier Science, Inc., New York.

American Journal of Cosmetic Surgery. Monthly publication of research articles.

Hair Transplant Forum International. Bimonthly publication of topics related to hair replacement surgery. Published by the International Society of Hair Replacement Surgery, Schaumberg, Illinois.

Hair Loss Journal Quarterly. The official consumer publication of the American Hair Loss Council, Chicago.

COMPUTER

Comptons On-line Encyclopedia, Comptons Learning Co., (Via) Prodigy ® Interactive Personal Service, 1992–Present.

ORGANIZATIONS

NATIONAL ALOPECIA AREATA FOUNDATION
710 C Street, Ste. 11
San Rafael, CA 94901
(415) 456-4644/FAX (415) 456-4644

AMERICAN HAIR LOSS COUNCIL
401 N. Michigan Ave.
Chicago, Illinois 60611
Consumer Hotline (800) 274-8717/FAX (312) 245-1080

AMERICAN ACADEMY OF COSMETIC SURGERY
401 North Michigan Road
Chicago, Illinois 60611
(312) 527-6713

AMERICAN SOCIETY FOR DERMATOLOGIC SURGERY
900 North Meacham Road
Schaumburg, Illinois 60173
(708) 330-9830/FAX (708) 330-0050

INTERNATIONAL SOCIETY FOR DERMATOLOGIC SURGERY
930 North Meacham Road
Schaumburg, Illinois 60173
(708) 330-9830/FAX (708) 330-0050

AMERICAN SOCIETY OF HAIR RESTORATION SURGEONS
401 North Michigan Road
Chicago, Illinois 60611
(312) 527-6713

INTERNATIONAL SOCIETY OF HAIR RESTORATION SURGERY
930 North Meacham Road
Schaumburg, Illinois 60173
(708) 330-9830/FAX (708) 330-0050

SPECIAL THANKS

Anthony Santangelo of AMS Designs, Chicago and President of American Hair Loss Council for his contributions on Hair Systems and Extensions.

Donte Cassese of For Men Only, Queens, N.Y. for his thirty-year retrospective on the hairpiece industry.

INDEX

R

S